Visual
Electrodiagnostic
Testing
a practical guide for the clinician

**This volume is one of the series
Handbooks in Ophthalmology
Edited by Walter S. Schachat**

Other books in this series include:

Klein and Katzin: Microsurgery of the Vitreous
Meltzer: Ophthalmic Plastic Surgery for the General Ophthalmologist
Thompson: Topics in Neuro-ophthalmology
Charles: Vitreous Microsurgery

Visual Electrodiagnostic Testing

a practical guide for the clinician

RONALD E. CARR, M.D.

Professor of Ophthalmology

IRWIN M. SIEGEL, Ph.D.

Professor of Research Ophthalmology

New York University Medical Center
New York, New York

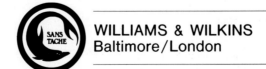

WILLIAMS & WILKINS
Baltimore/London

Copyright ©, 1982
Williams & Wilkins
428 East Preston Street
Baltimore, MD 21202, U.S.A.

Made in the United States of America

Library of Congress Cataloging in Publication Data

Carr, Ronald E.

   Visual electrodiagnostic testing.
   Bibliography: p.
   Includes index.
   1. Electrooculography. I. Siegel, Irwin M. II. Title [DNLM: 1. Electrodiagnosis. 2.
Eye diseases—Diagnosis. WW 143 C312v]
RE79.E39C37   617.7'1547   81-10330
ISBN 0-683-01462-5   AACR2
Composed and printed at the
Waverly Press, Inc.
Mt. Royal and Guilford Aves.
Baltimore, MD 21202, U.S.A.

Preface

Our colleagues and students have often asked us to recommend a practical manual discussing clinical applications of visual electrodiagnostic tests. We were able to refer them only to several articles and chapters that have appeared in journals or books, since no complete text addressed itself to the practice and application of electrical testing of the visual system. In spite of the great interest in ERG, EOG, and VEP testing and the ease with which these procedures could be performed, no comprehensive single treatment of clinico-diagnostic procedures was available. This book represents an attempt to somewhat remedy this situation.

A large portion of the text was suggested by questions put to us by the many fellows and residents who have worked at the New York University Medical Center Retinal Clinic. We are particularly indebted to the founders of the clinic, Dr. George Goodman and Professor Harris Ripps, for establishing testing techniques which emphasized the association between basic visual physiology and clinical diagnosis. We have endeavored to continue our own studies mindful of their innovative thinking and rigorous standards.

No large clinical center can be maintained without generous financial help. We would like to particularly acknowledge the many years of support from The National Eye Institute, The Retinitis Pigmentosa Foundation, Research to Prevent Blindness Inc., and the Fight-for-Sight.

The burden of preparing the text was greatly eased by the typing skills of Mrs. Sylvia Glasser and the photographic assistance of Mr. Walter Lentschner and Mr. Jack Brush.

Finally, we would like to thank the Chairman of the Ophthalmology Department, Dr. Goodwin M. Breinin, for his steadfast support of our clinical and research activities for over 20 years.

Contents

I. Basic Concepts and Methods

II. Clinical Section

III. Appendices

    I. Shielding and Filtering Requirements   102
    II. Amplifier Settings and ERG Calibration Procedures   103
    III. Strobe Flash Calibration   107
        A. Energy calibration of intensity   107
        B. Photometric calibration of the flash   107
    IV. Changing Flash-to-Eye Distance and Bright Flash Techniques   108
    V. Evaluating Photo- and Flash-Artifacts   109
    VI. The Use of Active 60-Hz Filters   109
B   **EOG: Technical Data** **110**
C   **Patient Safety Considerations** **111**
D   **Color Vision Testing** **113**
E   **Dark Adaptometry and Retinal Profiles** **118**

    References **120**
    Index **125**

Introduction

Electrical tests of visual function had their origins in the laboratory. Subsequent clinical applications were also confined to the laboratory since the equipment required was cumbersome and the instruments and patient usually had to be electrically shielded by large panels of copper screening. Because of these rarified beginnings, there evolved a small group of highly trained ophthalmologists with sufficient funds, technical assistance, and adequate time to perform tests which were thought much too difficult an undertaking for the busy clinician. This led to a great deal of misunderstanding in those who did not actually participate in performing the testing; it also resulted in disagreement as to the usefulness of such tests. There were some who felt that an electroretinogram (ERG), for example, would provide useful information for every disease of the retina while others claimed (with the same degree of certainty) that the ERG was much too diffuse a response to provide specific information about *any* retinal disease. After some years, the disputation between the "haves" and "have-nots" is less combative, and we can now more objectively delineate for the clinician which retinal diseases would benefit by ERG analysis and which would not.

While emphasis is placed on ERG recordings, electrical tests of a more specialized nature, such as the EOG and VEP, are also considered. Although the clinician may not perform these procedures himself, it is necessary to be aware of the circumstances in which they may be of diagnostic value.

Recent advances in electronic technology have resulted in many devices which are applicable for clinical ERG recording and other electrodiagnostic tests, procedures once thought to be properly performed only in the laboratory. Gone are the complex array of preamplifiers, driver amplifiers, elephantine pen recorders, and monstrous oscilloscopes. Many of these older instruments had to be modified and often required the help of an expert to be assembled into a working diagnostic system. In their place are self-contained, miniaturized units which accept the small voltage signals directly from the patient without accessory amplification, directly incorporate pen recording or oscilloscope display, and often have the capacity for signal averaging to detect very low voltage signals. In addition, few of the new instruments require shielding, which eliminates the need for large testing areas.

Clearly, the trend in instrumentation has been to provide the clinician with equipment that does not require highly trained engineers for its operation. Unfortunately, the ophthalmic literature has not sufficiently informed the clinician of this trend toward simplification. If anything, the electrodiagnostic studies of today appear more complex than those of several years ago. While it is true that more quantitative and meaningful studies are now being performed, it is no less true that the same equipment used in such studies can provide the busy clinician with an important diagnostic tool which he can operate himself either in his office or outpatient clinic.

The reader will quickly learn that electrical tests of visual function, far from being elitist procedures, are as convenient to perform on a patient as an ECG. We will try to emphasize that such tests can be considered routine diagnostic procedures which, along with the more commonly used techniques available to the practitioner, provide data which often reveal important aspects of a disease process. Electrical testing of the visual system also adds a dimension to ocular examination that was sadly lacking: a degree of objectivity.

Overawed, perhaps, by the beauty of the fundus landscape as viewed with an opthalmosocope, clinicians for the last 100 years have been prone to correlate visual dysfunction with those colorations, dots and flecks, and pigmentary changes of all shapes and sizes revealed by Helmholtz's ingenious invention. It was once suggested that if the chest wall were transparent and we could directly view the beating heart, cardiological diagnosis would not have arrived at the quantitative state it attained largely with the aid of indirect, objective, electrical measures of cardiac muscle tissue. The heart no doubt assumes a variety of surface coloration and morphological variation if we could view it during life. But we *cannot*, and we must decide whether a heart abnormality exists on a *functional* rather than an observational basis. Ophthalmoscopy is, of course, a most important part of any eye examination, and along with fundus photography provides invaluable diagnostic and prognostic information. All of us have been confronted with patients having serious visual difficulties with no obvious ophthalmoscopic changes. Conversely, we have observed the most bizarre-appearing fundi which are not associated with any detectable functional defect. While we are not suggesting that electrical testing will provide definitive clinical insight for either of these extreme instances, we have found, with intelligent application, that such testing does provide meaningful, quantitative data. For the clinician anxious to take the step from a predominantly descriptive approach to retinal disease, we will try to extend a helping hand. For some unfamiliar with the neurophysiological facts of visual function which are necessary for interpreting the electrical responses, we have begun the book with a few basic science sections. We urge those readers to whom such material is unfamiliar to take the time and read these chapters. More accurate diagnoses may be expected with an understanding of the workings of the retina and visual pathways.

Clinicians already at ease with neurophysiology may wish to use the manual simply as a technical guide to ERG and other types of electrical recordings. We have therefore detailed step by step procedures for those with no practical experience as well as for technicians who are being trained to do such testing under senior supervision.

We recognize that clinicians undertaking electrical testing will be using a variety of instrumentation. However, the basics of any of the commercially available electronic units do not differ significantly. Accordingly, we have aimed our technical sections toward a general understanding rather than presenting detailed minutiae of limited application. There are certain characteristics which electronic devices must possess in order to obtain recordings from the visual system. Too often, the clinician, because of his ignorance in this specialized area, will be coerced into buying a very sophisticated instrument package, which the salesman promises has "great potential." When confronted by a bewildering display of dials and knobs labeled in an unfamiliar jargon, the clinician may justifiably feel so intimidated that "routine electrical testing" may appear to him a bitter euphemism. We have placed emphasis on minimal instrumentation and maximal understanding of how such things as stimuli conditions, for example, can be varied to provide relevant clinical insights.

To preserve the concept of a true manual, the chapters are independent units which the clinician may refer to as the needs of the moment dictate. He may, for example, proceed immediately to the section on patient preparation or, to find out why a particular ERG record has a peculiar appearance, turn to the trouble-shooting section. We introduce the clinical section with *Diagnostic Guides*, which emphasizes the importance of the ERG findings for separating large groups of retinal diseases. Following this, detailed descriptions of disease categories are presented with their clinical, electrophysiological, and psychophysical results. For definitive diagnoses, there is no substitute for acquiring data from a battery of tests such as perimetry, dark adaptometry, and color vision. Only when the results of such ancillary procedures are known can one formulate a clear, unequivocal evaluation of some of the puzzling eye diseases which confront the clinician. The appendix contains outline procedures for obtaining some of these subjective data.

At the risk of injuring the feelings of those colleagues we do not mention, we have kept literature references in the body of the text to a minimum. We hope the interests of the clinician, in pursuing further knowledge of electrical testing, will be stimulated to seek out the selected books and journal references included at the end of the text.

Section One

Basic Concepts and Methods

1
Fundamentals of Electroretinography

It has been known for over 100 years that a flash of light will elicit a distinctive electrical response from the human eye—the electroretinogram (ERG). However, the step from laboratory curiosity to clinical application was not possible until the development of the contact lens in the 1940s.[1] The contact lens provided a stable, comfortable platform, which makes possible electrical continuity with the tear film of the cornea via a suitable conductive-cushioning fluid. Recently, modern electronic techniques have simplified the original recording procedures to the extent that an ERG is now a practical office and outpatient technique.

Little practical experience, however, is offered to most ophthalmology residents in training centers. Even though the ERG can be performed with rather simple apparatus, it is usually available only as a complex laboratory apparatus requiring the assistance of skilled technicians. The reader will soon learn that obtaining an ERG recording is no more difficult to perform than an electrocardiogram. In fact, the only substantial obstacle facing the clinician starting an ERG unit is in understanding the significance of the waveforms and how to apply this information to a variety of retinal diseases. A proper ERG protocol, incorporating light and dark adapted stimulus conditions, takes no more than 15 or 20 minutes. Yet, the data obtained can provide specific information about the functioning of particular neural portions of the retina.

In order for the ERG to be of practical diagnostic use, however, the clinician must have a clear idea of which structures in the retina are contributing to the response wave-form. This is accomplished by manipulating stimulus variables such as the flash intensity and color, frequency of flash presentation, and retinal adaptation. To this end, a brief primer of visual physiology for the clinician is presented.

THE DUPLEX RETINA AND ITS SIGNIFICANCE FOR THE ERG

There are several criteria which serve to distinguish the rods from the cones in the retina. Electron microscopy reveals obvious ultrastructural differences; photochemistry distinguishes between rod and cone photolabile pigments; and electrophysiology shows marked differences in the response of rod and cone membrane potentials to a flash of light. However, it was the disproportionate number of rods to cones (130 million to 7 million) and the unique distribution of the two receptor types in the retina that were noted first by early investigators. Microscopic preparations of the retina reveal great densities of cones in the foveal region which markedly decrease in number as one sections farther and farther from the foveola, until a region about 15° (4.5 mm) on either side of the foveola is reached, where the cone density continues to the periphery as a nearly constant but low value. Rods are excluded from the cone-rich foveola but precipitously rise in number proceeding away from this area, where they reach a maximum in the same area in which cone density levels off, i.e., 15° from the foveola. Rod density then decreases slightly from this peak value and maintains a steady, high value to the periphery.[2] Figure 1.1 incorporates estimates of rod and cone packing densities into an ophthalmoscopic view of the fundus.

Since the densities of rods and cones do not change greatly beyond 15° on either

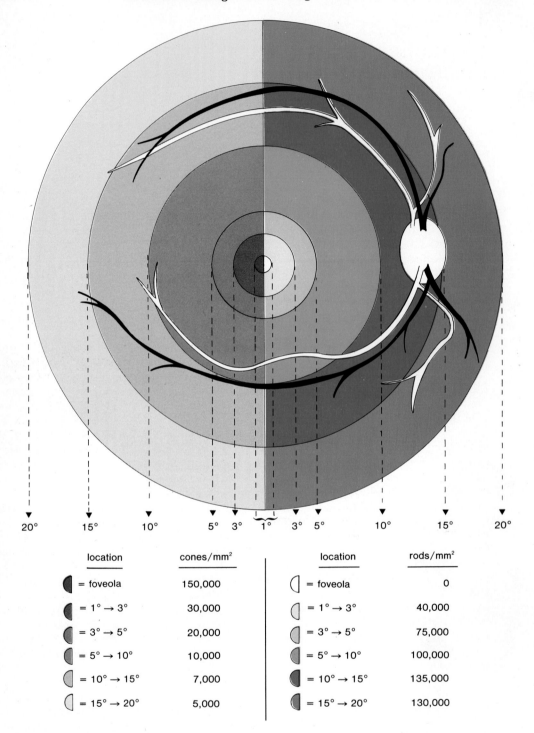

location	cones/mm²		location	rods/mm²
= foveola	150,000		= foveola	0
= 1° → 3°	30,000		= 1° → 3°	40,000
= 3° → 5°	20,000		= 3° → 5°	75,000
= 5° → 10°	10,000		= 5° → 10°	100,000
= 10° → 15°	7,000		= 10° → 15°	135,000
= 15° → 20°	5,000		= 15° → 20°	130,000

Figure 1.1 Retinal topographic construction showing population densities of cones (*red tones*) and rods (*blue tones*) superimposed on the fundus.

side of the foveola, they are not represented in the figure. Several points emerge, and some are more obvious than others. It is quite clear, for example, that if a retinal area had to be selected for testing the course of dark adaptation, an area rich in rods would be desirable. Figure 1.1 shows a high density of rods at 15° temporal retina, and it is this region that is usually chosen. The relatively small number of cones at 15° is still sufficient to yield measurements of cone adaptation also, though it is obviously the small foveola to which a test spot would be directed for a "pure" cone determination. The packing density at the exact center of the foveola is, in fact, calculated to be 150,000 cones/mm,^{2} so one might assume that the majority of retinal cones are indeed located in and around this very small central area. Nothing could be further from the truth! Computation shows that in spite of the high cone density in the foveola, it actually contains only about 9000 cones, i.e., less than 0.2% of the total cone population of the retina. Even considering the entire fovea (usually given as the central 5°), the number of cones in this larger area is still only a few percent of the total cone number. It is essential for the reader to appreciate that *the majority of cones lie outside the foveal region*. A practical consequence of this situation is that if the foveal area is damaged or diseased, ERG recordings which usually test total cone activity will appear perfectly normal. Conversely, when a decreased ERG cone response is obtained, an area considerably greater than the foveal diameter of 5° would have to have been affected. Underlying this finding is an important principle which will be emphasized many times in this manual: the clinical ERG is a summed or massed discharge of huge numbers of receptors. One of the great diagnostic virtues of the ERG is precisely that it does not "pay attention" to small retinal lesions. It provides the clinician with easily obtained, objective data which may indicate, for example, that a patient with decreased acuity and color vision deficit who shows a diminished ERG cone response does not merely have a foveal abnormality, but a generalized cone loss of the entire retina. One other

interesting fact is shown in Figure 1.1. The rod density increases so rapidly outside the fovea that only a few degrees away it is greater than the cone density. Even the so-called "macular area" is *rod* dominated!

Table 1.1 shows some of the functional properties of the rods and cones which enable the retina to demonstrate a remarkable degree of operating versatility. For many visual functions the two cell types work together, providing an enormous working range for the eye. The rod system, for example, is designed for the detection of very dim light stimuli, while the cones take over at moderate and high intensity conditions. When both systems are operating, the eye is sensitive to a billionfold change in illumination.

The dichotomy or "duplicity" of visual function under different illumination conditions derives from the anatomical, photochemical, and neural organizational differences between the rods and cones. Both cell types contain vitamin A-based light sensitive pigments. However, whereas the cones contain pigments sensitive to the blue, green, and red regions of the spectrum, the rods contain only a single blue-green sensitive pigment—rhodopsin. It should be pointed out that while the rod system can be stimulated by a broad range of colored lights, it cannot, by virtue of its particular neural network, signal color-coded information to the brain.

We can take advantage of the difference in rod and cone properties in order to record ERGs which will emphasize one system or the other. A dim blue light in the dark, for example, will stimulate predominantly the rods, whereas longer wave lengths, such as a deep red light or a brighter intensity, will stimulate, under light-adapted conditions, mostly cones. Similarly, taking advantage of the inability of rods to follow a fast-flickering light, we use a 30 per sec repetitive flash to isolate the cones.

THE APPEARANCE OF THE CLINICALLY RECORDED ERG WAVEFORM

Throughout this manual we have distinguished between a "clinical" ERG and the

Table 1.1
Functional Properties of Rods and Cones Which Enable the Retina to Demonstrate Remarkable Operating Versatility

	Rods	Cones
Sensitivity	To dim light	To bright light
Spatial resolution	Coarse visual acuity	Fine acuity
Temporal modulation	Only slow flicker (less than 10/sec)	Follow fast flicker
Maximal spectral sensitivity	Blue-green (500 nm)	Greenish-yellow (560 nm)
Rate of dark adaptation	Slow	Fast
Color vision	Absent	Present (requires at least 2 cone types)

more complex series of waves comprising the ERG recorded from animal preparations or from human subjects in rigorous laboratory circumstances. The distinction is a consequence of the recording conditions which, as a practical necessity, are used to obtain ERGs from naive, apprehensive and, often, uncooperative patients. Technical details of the actual instrument settings used and a complete discussion of the ERG waves are reserved for later chapters. For now, it suffices to state that there are only two major components of the clinically recorded ERG: the negative a-wave followed by the positive b-wave.

However, depending on the ambient room illumination, state of adaptation of the retina (i.e., whether it is relatively light or dark adapted), and the flash lamp intensity, the a- and b-waves achieve different amplitudes. For example, the largest ERG is obtained by using a bright white flash after dark-adapting the patient.

In Figure 1.2, the a- and b-waves are clearly delineated. The a-wave is measured from the base line downward to the very bottom of the negativity, and the b-wave is measured from the latter point upwards to the positive peak. Because the b-wave does not rise straight up, it is best to measure its amplitude by drawing a horizontal line from the a-wave notch and dropping a perpendicular from the estimated b-wave peak. The procedure is shown as a dashed line in Figure 1.2.

If the same bright flash is delivered to an eye which was light adapted (i.e., in moderate room illumination), the a- and b-wave amplitudes are reduced to about 30% of the dark adapted values. This is shown in Figure 1.3.

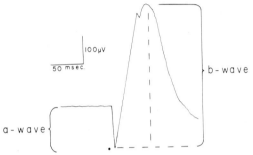

Figure 1.2 Typical form of a clinically recorded dark-adapted (scotopic) ERG in response to a flash of high intensity. A flash presentation is indicated in this and all succeeding figures by a *solid circle*. The a-wave amplitude is measured from the preflash base line down to the lowest negative excursion of the trace, and the b-wave amplitude is measured from this point to the highest positive peak. The calibration lines allow computation of duration or peak times (in milliseconds = msec and amplitude in microvolts = μV).

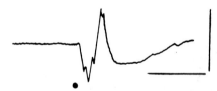

Figure 1.3 A light-adapted retina produces, in response to a bright flash, a fast, brisk (photopic) ERG. Note that the response is considerably smaller and quite different in shape than the scotopic ERG (Fig. 1.2), even though the flash intensities are identical. Calibration lines denote 50 msec (horizontal) and 200 μV (vertical).

Note that the entire wave-form has a shorter duration and the b-wave a more pointed appearance than in the dark-adapted ERG. From the previous discussion, it should be clear that the change from dark to light adaptation has shifted the operating characteristics of the retina from the slower but more sensitive rod system to the faster, less sensitive, cone system. Since the cones are substantially fewer in number than rods (about 1 cone to 17 rods), and are intrinsically 10 times less sensitive (see Fig. 2.3), the amplitude of the cone ERG is accordingly smaller.

Regardless of the state of retinal adaptation during recording, however, it should be obvious from Fig. 1.2 and 1.3 that the b-wave is the dominant component of the clinical ERG. In fact, if one directs a weak flash of light to the dark-adapted, eye no a-wave is detectable. As shown in Figure 1.4, only a slowly developing b-wave of low amplitude appears under such circumstances.

Clearly, the relative contributions of the a- and b-waves can be markedly altered by changing the stimulus flash intensity and the state of adaptation of the retina. A fuller explanation of why these variables are important is taken up in the section dealing with the origin of the ERG responses. However, one must not conclude from the information given thus far that the a-wave is somehow a cone-derived potential. In fact, it will be seen that the rod and cone systems both contribute to the a- and b-waves.

It should be clear at this point that by applying flashes of different intensity to the dark- or light-adapted retina, changing the flash repetition rate, or changing the color of the flash with suitable filters, we can selectively emphasize rod or cone activity.

In summary, to record an ERG that reflects predominantly cone function, one would:

1. Have the testing environment moderately illuminated to maintain a light-adapted state.
2. In addition to a single high intensity flash, use a flicker rate of 20 to 30 per second.

Figure 1.5 illustrates a typical flicker-following response of the light-adapted eye.

Note the slightly larger amplitude ERG to the first flash in the figure. The rods probably contribute a small amount to this initial response but cannot recover fast enough to affect subsequent responses.

To record an ERG that reflects predominantly rod activity, one would:

1. Dark adapt the patient for at least 10 to 15 minutes.
2. Use a low intensity flash stimulus, preferably with a blue filter in front of the flash lamp.
3. Use a single high intensity flash to obtain some idea of the full voltage generated by the rod-dominated dark adapted retina.

SCATTERED LIGHT AND THE CLINICAL ERG

Early investigators noted that an intense flash focused to a very small spot on the retina produced a much greater ERG response than expected.[3] In fact, if the image of the flash was confined only to the optic nerve head, an ERG as large as one from a functioning area of retina was generated. This finding has great significance for the

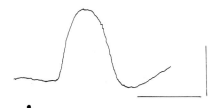

Figure 1.4   ERG response of the dark-adapted eye to a dim blue flash. Wave-form characteristics typical for this stimulus condition are the relatively long time-to-peak of the b-wave, the smooth rounded appearance of the b-wave, and the absence of an a-wave. Calibration: 80 msec (*horizontal line*) and 200 μV (*vertical line*).

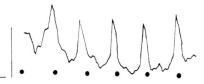

Figure 1.5   A repetitive high intensity flash presentation (shown here at about 30 times/second) produces the so-called flicker following response. For each flash (indicated by the *black circles*) a well-defined ERG is developed. Calibration lines indicate 50 msec and 200 μV.

clinician performing electroretinography. A flash bright enough to obtain an ERG will scatter light onto regions of the retina far from the area upon which the flash is directly imaged. Since the ERG is a massed electrical response, the recording electrode summates potentials generated by all activated regions of the retina—those weakly stimulated by scatter as well as those areas directly stimulated. Therefore, it is necessary at the very least to use a diffuser over the flash lamp to provide more even illumination on the directly stimulated portions of the retina. If a flash lamp with a 6-inch circular diffuser is placed 16 inches from the eye, it subtends about 20° at the cornea. This in turn directly stimulates a 30-mm^2 area of retina and indirectly scatters light over very large retinal areas. While the overall luminance is not spread uniformly enough across the retina to accurately measure ERG latencies (discussed in Chapter 6), this configuration is sufficient to produce reliable ERGs with amplitudes great enough for most clinical purposes.

2

Analysis of the ERG Components

It is clear from the previous discussion that the amplitude and wave-forms of the clinically recorded electroretinogram (ERG) undergo many changes as the flash intensity, state of retinal adaptation, and other stimulus conditions are varied. To intelligently evaluate a recording, we must, therefore, be able to answer the following questions.

1. Do the amplitudes and wave-form characteristics fall within a range of "normal"? If not, what does such an abnormality signify? This query relates to the standardization of the ERG recordings and is taken up in Chapter 5.

2. Do we know where in the retina the a- and b-waves have their origin, and which neural elements generate them? If we can make this identification, then we may infer from the ERG which layers of the retina are involved in a particular disease.

It has been known for many years that the ERG wave-form is an envelope of electrical activity, deriving from different retinal regions. The individual components making up the composite are potentials of different polarity, amplitude, duration, and latency. Therefore, while each wave will be seen to have quite simple characteristics, the sum total may have a complicated appearance. Nonetheless, for diagnostic purposes it is essential to know which component of the ERG complex is responsible for a change in the overall wave-form. One of the classic ways to demonstrate how the ERG develops is to fractionate (subtract out) from the overall wave-form the largest contribution—the b-wave.

There are several ways to accomplish the fractionation, but one of the more ob-vious techniques is to take advantage of the fact that the inner and outer retinal layers have separate vascular supplies. In an animal preparation, for example, a metal rod can be inserted through the vitreous cavity and pressed against the central retinal artery as it emerges from the surface of the optic disc.[4] Alternatively, the optic nerve containing the artery can be ligated.[5] The inner retinal layers, up to and including the inner plexiform layer, become immediately anoxic after either procedure, and the b-wave rapidly diminishes, producing an ERG which becomes more and more negative in appearance. Figure 2.1 shows schematically how such fractionation affects ERGs recorded in the dark-adapted eye using bright flashes.

Note that as the b-wave disappears, the character of the tracing becomes negative, and what finally remains is a deep, sustained negative-going wave. The latter potential, therefore, must derive from activity primarily generated in the photoreceptor region, since this layer is still nourished by an intact choroidal circulation. This isolated negative wave is, in fact, called the *receptor potential* of the retina. By inference, then, the b-wave derives from the inner retinal layers. However, a great variety of studies, including the early one by Karpe,[6] have shown that ganglion cell activity *does not contribute* to the standard clinical ERG. Therefore, the b-wave that is recorded in most clinical situations is probably generated by structures in the mid-retinal layers. Some of the recent work on b-wave origin is discussed in Chapter 3. Thus the clinical ERG is seen to be the summation of a negative receptor potential and a positive wave arising from the mid-retinal layers.

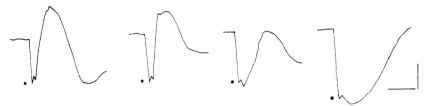

Figure 2.1 Fractionation of the ERG by anoxia. The complete ERG wave-form (shown at the left) loses its positive b-wave component over a period of several minutes as the central retinal artery is closed off. Note that as the b-wave diminishes an underlying negative potential (the receptor potential) of large amplitude is gradually unmasked. It is a portion of the leading edge of the receptor potential that one denotes as the "a-wave" in response to a bright flash in clinical records. Calibration lines indicate 50 msec and 200 μV.

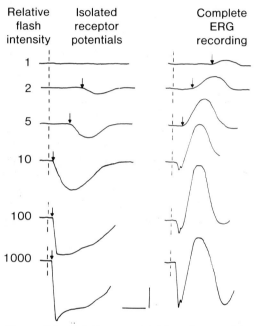

Figure 2.2 Relative sensitivities of a- and b-wave responses can be compared by first obtaining ERG recordings to a series of graded intensity flashes (right hand column) and repeating the run after experimentally isolating the receptor potential (left hand column). The greater sensitivity of the b-wave is indicated by the fact that at the lowest stimulus intensity (top row) a small b-wave is elicited while the same flash evokes no detectable receptor potential. The figure also demonstrates why the a-wave (which is the leading edge of the receptor potential) does not appear in the complete ERG response to low intensities. Because the receptor potential is generated so slowly at low intensities it is completely masked by the earlier appearing b-wave. Only at high flash intensities (10) does the receptor potential appear early enough to be detected. Calibration: 40 msec. (horizontal) and 200 μV (vertical line).

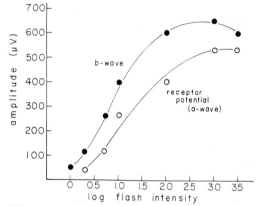

Figure 2.3 Tracings of Figure 2.2 are shown here in graph form. This type of representation is a voltage vs. intensity (V log I) plot for the a- and b-wave response amplitudes to a graded series of flash intensities. The greater sensitivity of the b-wave to a flash of any intensity is particularly obvious at the lower values.

What we label as the "a-wave" in the complete ERG recording can now be identified as only the leading edge of the receptor potential. Note also that the amplitude of this leading edge is larger when the receptor potential is isolated (last trace, Fig. 2.1). What has happened is that the b-wave has masked the receptor potential and has cut short its full development.

Considering that the chain of electrical events runs from the photoreceptors to the bipolars and finally to the ganglion cells, it might seem odd that a second order neural change such as the b-wave could successfully obscure a primary one (the a-wave). However, one needs only to consider the relative sensitivities of the isolated receptor potential and the b-wave to account for this unusual interaction. If one were to isolate the receptor potential using the arterial occlusion technique described above, and test the sensitivity of the dark-adapted eye with flashes of increasing intensity, one obtains records similar to those shown in the left column of Figure 2.2. On the right of Figure 2.2 is shown ERG recordings to the same series of flashes. By comparing the amplitudes of the two different responses to the low intensity flashes (first few rows), it becomes clear that the b-wave is far more sensitive. For example, at flash intensity 2, the receptor potential is barely recordable while the b-wave is quite large. Note also that the *absolute latency* (interval between the flash and the response onset) of the receptor potential, is longer than the b-wave latency at these low intensities. In fact, it is only when the flashes become bright that the receptor potential responds fast enough to get its leading edge (the a-wave) included as part of the ERG. It is only after intensity 10, when both waves are included in the complete ERG, that the ERG appears as a complex interaction of two opposite-going potentials. Little wonder that it has been decided, for clinical purposes, that when both a- and b-waves are present, we measure the b-wave amplitude from its peak to the trough (most negative-going portion) of the a-wave.

Figure 2.3 shows in graphic form the data depicted in Figure 2.2 and illustrates the dramatic differences in amplitude and sensitivity between the receptor potential and b-wave over a large range of intensities. The decrease in amplitude of the b-wave for high intensities is attributable to the fact that this measure begins (arbitrarily) from the a-wave trough, which itself is steadily increasing in amplitude as the receptor potential responds to the brighter flashes.

One final point about a- and b-wave interactions. It is frequently asked: "What are the *isolated b-wave* characteristics?" "why cannot the b-wave be studied apart from the other ERG components in a manner similar to that used to investigate the a-wave?" The answer is that any of the possible fractionation techniques, such as making the choroidal vessels anoxic or applying toxic chemicals to obliterate the photoreceptors will simpy eliminate the *entire* ERG. If the first neuron in the chain of electrical events is eliminated, then subsequent events also cease.

3

Physiology of ERG Activity

The discussion in the previous chapter will provide the clinician with sufficient information about ERG activity to satisfy most diagnostic inquiries. However, there is a new body of information concerning the physiology of the cells contributing to ERG potentials which should not be overlooked. This detailed understanding of how the potentials are generated makes the ERG a more precise indicator of disease location in the retina, as well as providing further clues to the etiology of disease processes themselves. It has been through microelectrode penetration studies of individual retinal cells that the most recent data on the ERG components developed.

Each major cell type in the retina has been penetrated by a microelectrode and recordings obtained in response to a flash of light. Typically, the electrode is filled with electrolyte dye and driven through the retina, micron by micron, while stimulating the retina with light. After an experiment, the dye is electrically forced into the cell, the tissue is fixed, and the cell is anatomically identified as to type. Following are some of the findings derived from only a few of these remarkable studies.

In the dark there is a continuous electrical current maintaining the receptors at a relatively positive level. The sodium ion is responsible for this "dark current"[7]. As indicated in Figure 3.1A, the sodium leaves the inner segment of the receptor (the current "source") and enters the outer segment (the current "sink").

The high flux of Na^+ leaving the inner segments and entering the outer segment of the receptor is indicated by the dark arrows in Figure 3.1A. When light is absorbed, the sodium channels of the recep- tor membrane are blocked, presumably by calcium released from the surface of outer segment lamellae. The light-induced decrement in Na^+ flow is depicted in Figure 3.1B as *dashed lines*. Oscilloscope recordings are placed next to the dark-adapted receptor and next to the one which has just received a flash. The negative (hyperpolarizing) response seen in Figure 3.1B is, in fact, the receptor potential. It should be mentioned, as a final qualifier, that the receptor potential itself is *not* a "pure" response but contains both a true receptor component—the initial portion—derived from the receptor, and a later slower portion, which probably originates from glial cell activity.[8]

Light-induced electrical changes in the receptor membrane regulate the release of chemical transmitters at the photoreceptor synaptic terminal. This, in turn, produces a membrane potential change in the second neuron, the bipolar cells.[9] Figures 3.2A and B depict microelectrode penetration into two classes of bipolar cell—one which depolarizes (Fig. 3.2A), and the other (Fig. 3.2B), which hyperpolarizes in response to a flash of light.[10] We usually speak of the ERG b-wave as originating "in the midretinal layers." Are the bipolar cell potentials, in fact, the ERG b-wave? The bipolar cells, like the receptors, are radially oriented, and so the remote electrodes could very well sense a massed bipolar discharge. However, as shown by microelectrode recordings, the temporal characteristics of the bipolar wave-form are quite different from those of b-wave. More important is the fact that half the bipolars depolarize and the other half hyperpolarize when excited. The algebraic summation of these events would yield a zero

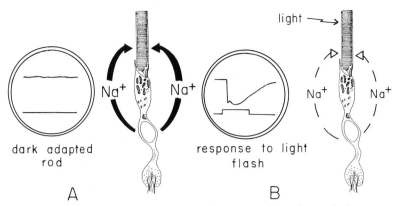

Figure 3.1 An electrical current, mediated by sodium ions, flows from the inner segment to the outer segment of the photoreceptor. In the dark, the current density is highest, indicated by the *heavy arrows* in A. The dark sodium current maintains the receptor in a depolarized state. When the receptor is exposed to light, the sodium current decreases, as shown in B, and the membrane hyperpolarizes. It is this slow negative change in photoreceptor activity that is referred to as the receptor potential.

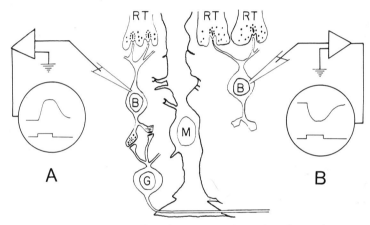

Figure 3.2 Recording from a bipolar cell with a penetrating microelectrode may result in either a depolarizing potential (A) or a hyperpolarizing potential (B). Both types of membrane changes shift the potassium concentration of the intracellular milieu. One theory holds that the Mueller cells then respond to the K⁺ changes, and it is this electrical potential which is remotely recorded as the ERG b-wave. *RT,* receptor terminal; *M,* Mueller cell; *B,* bipolar cell; *G,* ganglion cell.

potential (insofar as an ERG electrode could determine), and *no* potential is then likely to be detected. Figure 3.2 also shows a large glial structure, the Mueller cell, the proximal terminal of which forms the internal limiting membrane. Its distal end forms specialized appositions onto several receptor inner segments which, when viewed across the retina, comprise the so-called external limiting membrane. Like glia in other nervous tissue, the Mueller cells behave as potassium-sensitive elec-

trodes. That is, their membranes change potential as a function of the concentration of extracellular K^+.

The original model proposed that as bipolar cells of either type are excited, the extracellular concentration of K^+ increases. Mueller cells sense this change in K^+ concentration and respond by a membrane depolarization.[11] Recent studies indicate that while the ERG b-wave derives much of its origin from Mueller cells,[12] it is not its sole derivation and other (uniden-

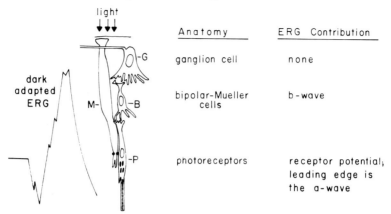

Figure 3.3 The clinically recorded ERG in response to a diffuse flash is a composite of waveforms derived from different layers of the retina. Photoreceptors generate the a-wave (which is the leading edge of the receptor potential), and midretinal layer structures produce the b-wave via Mueller cell activation.

tified) neural structures participate in its development.[13] Nonetheless, the facts for clinical ERG work are clear:

(1) The b-wave does originate, probably in an indirect manner from neuroglial structures in the midlayers of the retina.

(2) The b-wave is a very accurate measure of retinal sensitivity and, using appropriate procedures, may be used to determine such functions as dark adaptation, spectral sensitivity, and flicker fusion functions.

The reason why b-wave activity so overwhelms receptor potential activity is that a great deal of neural facilitation or "convergence" takes place in the midlayers of the retina and produces a sizeable amplification or "gain" of potential. Consider for a moment that there are about 130 million receptors in the retina and only one million nerve fibers exiting via the optic nerve. The receptors, for the most part, behave as independent detectors while the bipolars (via the lateral interaction of horizontal cells) are major benefi-

ciaries of the funneled discharge, and subsequently produce sufficient increase in extracellular K^+ which results (via the Muller, i.e., glial cells) in a very large change in potential.

Figure 3.3 is a summary of the ERG components covered thus far. Note that the lateral interacting horizontal and amacrine cells are not shown. This is not because they are unimportant. Quite to the contrary, their functions are most essential for visual processing, but they make no obvious contribution to the generation of the clinically recorded (flash) ERG.

The cascade sequence of electrical signaling is made clear in the figure: photoreceptors—bipolars—ganglion cells—optic nerve. It should now be obvious that the ERG reflects only a limited portion of activity that takes place in the visual pathway. Without intact ganglion cells and a normal optic nerve, the retinal signals do not reach the higher centers and we cannot see—despite the presence of a normal ERG.

4

Patient Preparation and ERG Protocols

Regardless of the system of recording employed—paper polygraph or oscilloscope display—the interfacing of patient and instrument remains the same. This is shown schematically in Figure 4.1.

Before the particulars of preparing the patient are given, some general points must be stated.

Instrumentation. The electronic system used for electroretinogram (ERG) recording may require copper screening around the patient to reduce 60-Hz interference (Hz = cycles per second). The reader should consult the section in this manual (Appendix A) dealing with this point before beginning a recording with unfamiliar equipment and before purchasing an apparatus with which to perform the ERG, although most of the commercial ERG instruments incorporate the appropriate electronic requisites.

Recording Environment. The room in which the recording is to be done should be moderately illuminated and also be relatively light proof when the room lights are extinguished. If the light adapted ERG from a normal eye recorded with the highest flash intensity appears small (less than 75 μV), then the ambient light may be too bright (see Fig. 5.1). Generally, this ERG response should be from 100 to 200 μV and the time flash to peak (implicit latency) should be 25 ± 3 msec. Room illumination should be suitably adjusted to produce a response falling in this range. If a ganzfeld bowl is used, the room is darkened and the bowl illumination is adjusted to produce a brisk-looking photopic response to a bright flash.

Patient Position. If possible, we recommend that the patient be placed in a supine

position for the recording. If a table is not available, a lounge recliner chair will suffice. An ordinary examining chair can also be used if its back folds back far enough. In the supine position, the patient is more relaxed, and the clinician can more conveniently prepare the patient for the test. For infants and young children especially, supine recording is essential.

PATIENT PREPARATION

A step-by-step procedure for preparing a patient is given in the series of photographs in Figures 4.2 and 4.3. The patient should be briefly told the nature of the test and what will be expected. We have found that analogy of the ERG to the electrocardiogram (which most patients have experienced) provides a suitable example. Attention should be drawn to the flash lamp (or fixation point in the diffuser bowl) and a demonstration of the flash should be given. Before the contact lens electrode is inserted, the patient's lids can be lightly held open while the examiner explains that this sensation, i.e., "a little pressure against the lids," is all that will be experienced. Mention should be made that a contact lens will be placed on the eye (not into the eye) in order to make the recording. A drop of topical anesthetic is now instilled in the eye to be tested (Fig. 4.2A). While waiting for corneal anesthesia, the following steps can be done. A small area on the center of the forehead is cleaned with an alcohol sponge and then rubbed vigorously dry (Fig. 4.2B). A dab of saline jelly (or electrode paste) is rubbed into the center of the cleaned area; the reference

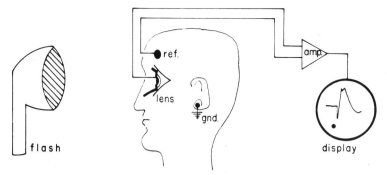

Figure 4.1 The basic components required to record a clinical ERG are shown. Not shown is the flash synchronized electrical signal which indicates where on the record the flash appears, seen as a *black circle* in the display inset.

electrode with a small amount of jelly is then pressed firmly onto the prepared area and taped into place (Fig. 4.2C). The dab of conducting paste should be applied, even when using disposable reference electrodes (of the ECG type). A ground electrode is attached to the ear or wrist using a squeeze clip or ECG grounding plate, respectively, in the manner suggested for the reference electrode (Fig. 4.2, D and E).

It should be mentioned that the Burian-Allen type contact lens electrode is available in both the "monopolar" form, as illustrated in Figure 4.3 and in "bipolar" form, which means that the speculum portion is coated with a conducting material; the palpebral conjuctiva therefore serves as a reference point. The bipolar electrode thus has two leads, one from the contact lens and the other from the lid reference. If this lens is used, no forehead reference is required. Despite its convenience, however, this type of electrode can produce great variability in the recorded ERG amplitudes (e.g., shorting between the cornea and lids via the tears and wetting solution may result in a decreased ERG amplitude). After trying both types, it is our feeling that a monopolar (single lead) contact lens with a separate forehead reference point should be used. If a bipolar electrode gives unsatisfactory results, it may be converted to monopolar by simply clipping the lead attached to the speculum and using a separate forehead reference, as shown in Figure 4.2.

We must stress that the location to

which the reference electrode is affixed is a *recording* point, and proper placement of this electrode on the forehead is essential for good quality recordings.

By now the cornea should be anesthetized. One more drop of anesthetic is placed in the eye, and contact lens insertion may then begin. As shown in Figure 4.3B, the examiner holds the lens speculum between the thumb and the first finger. The patient is asked to look towards his feet. The examiner then gently lifts the upper lid with his free hand and inserts the flange beneath the upper lid. The patient is then asked to look up, and the lower flange of the lens is tucked under the lower lid (Fig. 4.3C). Note that the speculum handle of the lens remains in an inferior position.

Small pieces of tape can be used to tack the leads of the reference and contact lens electrode down to the forehead and cheek. In case the patient inadvertently moves his head, the adhesive tape will help prevent the electrodes from pulling loose. If the patient has a very wide palpebral fissure or very flaccid lids, the electrodes may pop out of the eye or rotate. If this occurs, you may want to position the electrode with the handle pointing toward the temporal canthus. As a last resort, try lightly taping the lids so they close over the flanges of the lens speculum.

The three electrode leads (ground, reference, and contact lens) go to their respective openings in the input receptacle. If the reference and contact lens are reversed, an upside-down ERG will result. If

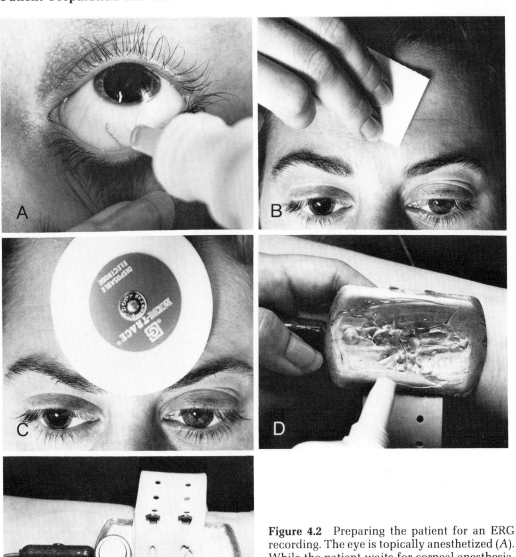

Figure 4.2 Preparing the patient for an ERG recording. The eye is topically anesthetized (*A*). While the patient waits for corneal anesthesia, the forehead is prepared to receive the reference electrode with an alcohol sponge and is briskly dried with a tissue (*B*). A disposable-type adhesive-backed reference electrode is affixed to the prepared forehead area (*C*), and the patient is grounded using either an ECG wrist plate dabbed with conducting paste (*D & E*) or an ear clip.

either the active electrode lead or the inactive reference is mistakenly plugged into ground, a flat base line (shorted input) or a very noisy trace will appear.

If a multichannel polygraph is being used, make sure you know which pen is recording the right eye and which the left.

To avoid confusion, routinely reserve the uppermost channel for the right eye and the next lowest channel for the left.

The flash lamp or diffuser bowl should now be swung into position above the patient's face (Fig. 4.3E). If a bowl is used the patient's face goes into the opening as

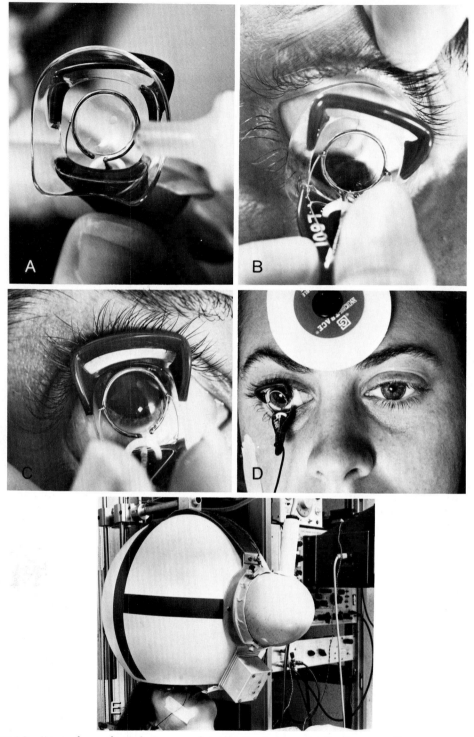

Figure 4.3 Corneal anesthesia being complete, the final steps of patient preparation may proceed. A drop of any tear substitute containing methylcellulose is placed on the posterior surface of the contact lens of the eye electrode (*A*). The examiner grasps the handle of the electrode between thumb and first finger. The patient is told to look down, and the superior portion of the electrode speculum is slipped under the upper lid (*B*). The patient is then asked to look up, and the examiner, still holding the handle of the electrode, inserts the inferior portion of the speculum behind the lower lid (*C*). The final positions of the reference and active eye electrode are shown in *D*. The ganzfeld bowl is then lowered into position over the patient's face (*E*). If a strobe lamp is used, it is placed about 1 foot above the patient's face and is centered over the chin so that the patient's eyes are directed slightly downward to reduce forehead wrinkling.

shown in the figure. When direct strobe lamp stimulation is used, position the lamp about 12 inches from the face and tilted towards the eyes. This prevents forehead wrinkling and is a more comfortable gaze position for the patient.

At this point, demonstrate to the patient what will be expected of him by flashing the lamp at a low intensity. Ask him to be as relaxed as possible—no forehead wrinkling or jaw tightening. Explain that squeezing the eyes before or during the flash will prevent recording and that he should try not to blink during the flash. While it is true that most patients cannot do this, the ERG is usually generated before a blink develops so that a blink artifact will in most cases follow the fully developed ERG.

A test recording should be made to ensure that all connections have been properly attended to and also to establish further patient cooperation. The clinician can now proceed with the actual recording.

ERG RECORDING PROTOCOLS

Since flash intensities will often be different, depending on the photostimulator unit used, we have purposely not specified in the following protocols exactly what is meant by "low" or "high" intensities in photometric terms. In Chapter 1, it was mentioned that the ERG amplitude and wave form characteristics themselves are excellent guides to the strength of the flash intensity. Thus a "high" intensity flash under photopic conditions produces a relatively small amplitude, short latency ERG with sharply peaked a- and b-waves. After 10 minutes of dark adaptation, a "low" intensity white or blue flash produces an ERG without a detectable (or very small) a-wave and a softly rounded b-wave.

Photostimulator and Flashes of Different Intensities

Since most ERG workers in the United States use one particular flash unit—the Grass PS-22 Photostimulator (Fig. 4.4)—a few words about the intensity settings of this instrument are appropriate. The intensity dial has five positions labeled in octaves: 1, 2, 4, 8, and 16. A designation of S_{16} white refers to the highest, unattenuated lamp strength, while an S_1 blue flash is the lowest intensity transmitted through a blue filter, such as the one supplied by the Grass Company. It should not be assumed that the doubling scale on the dial refers to a doubling of flash intensity; the S_{16} setting does not yield a flash 16 times brighter than the S_1 setting. Actual photometric flash values will be discussed in Appendix A, section III. We consider a S_1 flash as "low" and a S_{16} as "high" intensity.

Every clinician who gains some expertise doing ERGs will eventually design his own protocol. Keeping in mind the great number of variables which can be manipulated, the protocol can evolve into a long and detailed examination. Based on our own clinical experiences, however, we have learned that only a few stimulus conditions are required for most diagnostic purposes. It is also important to remember that the cornea does not tolerate most forms of contact lens electrodes for extensive periods of time. No patient should spend more than one-half hour with a contact lens electrode resting on the cornea. The protocols suggested below should take no more than 15 to 20 minutes to administer.

Protocol 1

A. Light-adapted ERG (performed under moderate room or bowl illumination)
  1. High intensity single flashes. One or two responses are sufficient.
  2. A short burst of high intensity flicker (30/second). Often a patient's eye blink or lid sqeeze prevents no more than a small segment of the "flicker" response to be recorded. However, under most circumstances, only four or five flicker responses are necessary to confirm normal values for this stimulus condition.
B. Dark-adapted ERG—after 10 minutes of complete darkness
  1. Low intensity (S_1) flash with a blue filter
  2. Low intensity (S_1) white flash

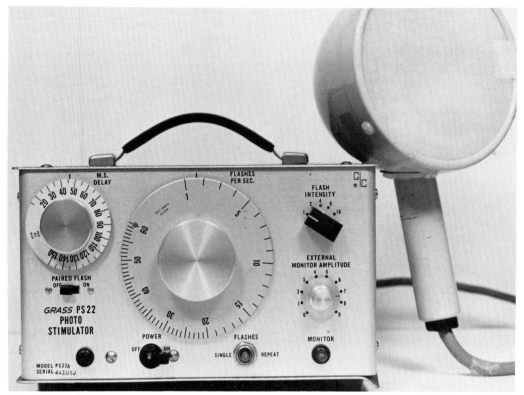

Figure 4.4　The photostimulator provides flashes of five different intensities. Although the flash intensity numbers are shown in multiples of 2, this does not correspond to a photometric intensity doubling. Repetitive flash rates are set with the center dial. The instrument provides a flash synchronized artifact, the height of which is related to the intensity setting. An external monitor control permits adjustment of the stimulus artifact and is used if the synchronized pulses are too small or too large.

3. High intensity (S_{16}) white flash

When delivering high intensity flashes to the dark-adapted eye, remember to allow at least 30 seconds to elapse between flashes. Continuous flashing in the dark will light adapt the retina and desensitize it, producing smaller ERG responses.

Protocol 2

A. Dark-adapted ERG

Patient is dark adapted by means of a patch or is left in darkness for 15 or 20 minutes (or longer) *without* a contact lens on the eye. The lens is inserted in the eye just prior to recording, using dim red illumination.

1. Single low intensity blue flash
2. Low intensity white flash
3. High intensity white flash

B. Light-adapted ERG

The room lights or bowl illumination are turned on, and the patient is given about a minute or so to become comfortable at the new level of illumination.

1. Single high intensity flash
2. Burst of 30/second high intensity flashes

There are several advantages to Protocol 1. The patient is given a chance to acclimate to the procedure with a lens in his eye. The 30/second flicker stimulus is bright enough to wipe out the effects of previous light adaptation (e.g., from ophthalmoscopy fundus photography), producing in effect a "standard" light adaptation. Thus each patient goes into the 10-minute period of dark adaptation with about the same level of retinal sensitivity. Finally, the fact that protocol 1 is overall a shorter procedure makes the most efficient use of patient-examiner time.

Protocol 2 allows a long period of dark adaptation without the risk of corneal trauma. Therefore, it certainly should be used for those patients suspected of being congenitally night-blind, and it is especially useful in those forms of nyctalopia, such as Oguchi's disease or fundus albipunctatus, which require 2 or 3 hours of darkness for return of retinal sensitivity.

Protocol 3

Determining Amplitude vs. Intensity Functions

If the relation between b-wave amplitude and flash intensity is to be determined (the so-called V log I relation), a precisely graded series of flash intensities is required. In order to provide a series of flashes which quantitatively differ from each other by a known amount, one should place neutral density filters (Kodak 96) in front of the flash lamp. Starting with a 4.0 density filter over the S_{16} flash, a barely detectable response may be obtained from the dark adapted eye. The next response is recorded using the same flash setting (S_{16}) but with a 3.5 density filter. With a 3.0 density filter the flash is now 10 times brighter than it was with a 4.0, and the ERG amplitude is correspondingly larger. A 2.0 density filter produces a flash 100 times brighter, and so on. It is important to wait about 1 minute between flashes at the higher intensities. Thus it is possible to obtain a 10,000-fold range in equal logarithmic intervals using neutral density filters of appropriate value (as shown in Fig. 2.3). Smaller intensity intervals may be produced by interpolating 0.5 or 0.3 density filters anywhere in the sequence.

ABBREVIATED PROTOCOLS

There are many circumstances which force the examiner to forego a complete protocol and simply try to obtain as much information as possible in a short period of time. Anxious patients or uncooperative children, for example, will be better handled by a shorter ERG procedure. We suggest that a single bright flash and a high intensity flicker recording be immediately obtained on *all patients*. The room lights are then turned off and the same (single) high intensity flash is delivered to the eye about every 30 seconds. Normal eyes will respond by a steady increase in a- and b-wave amplitudes each time a flash is given. Large increments in response, even over a *short* (1- to 2-minute) period of dark adaptation, are indicative of a functional scotopic mechanism. On the other hand, lack of scotopic increments after several minutes in the dark are consistent with a defective rod system, such as a tapetoretinal degeneration or congenital nightblindness.

5

ERG Standardization

ESTABLISHING NORMAL ERG VALUES

The essence of ERG diagnosis is the ability to determine whether or not a particular response is normal. It should be obvious, however, that criteria of normality such as amplitude and wave-form characteristics are as much dependent on the flash stimulus conditions as on patient variables such as pupil size, clarity of the ocular media, fundus coloration, and age. In order to establish a range of normal ERG values, therefore, it is necessary (among other things) to compare any given patient against a sizeable group of normal subjects of about the same age tested under identical conditions.

The clinician need only keep his recording conditions reasonably constant in order to attain diagnostically useful data. Nonetheless, it is absolutely necessary to run a group of normals (greater numbers ensure a higher degree of confidence) and establish a range of amplitude values which can be used for patient diagnosis. About 20 normal patients, aged 18 to 50 years, is a reasonable sample. High myopes, even those with good correctable vision, should *not* be included in this standard group. Younger patients have larger ERGs, and older subjects will have slightly smaller ones. Some typical light- and dark-adapted values are given in Table 5.1 and are illustrated in Figures 1.2, 1.3, and 1.4. Remember that the amplitude of the ERG b-wave is also sensitive to recording variables such as ambient room illumination, length of dark adaptation, flash-to-eye distance, and, of course, intensity of the flash. Therefore, it is necessary to establish a normal range consistent with the testing environment.

DETERMINING BACKGROUND ILLUMINATION FOR LIGHT-ADAPTED ERG RECORDINGS

Simply put, the ambient illumination (background) should be bright enough to ensure the clinician that the recorded response is generated primarily by the cones. To understand the problem, assume that extreme levels of background illumination are used, i.e., too dim and too bright. If the ambient light on the retina is low, the rods are capable of participating and interfering

Table 5.1
Typical Light- and Dark-adapted Values

Flash intensity	Light-adapted b-wave amplitudes (μV)	Dark-adapted b-wave amplitudes (μV)
Low*	20–40 (not commonly done)	100–200 (white) 75–150 (blue)
High*	80–150	300–500

* Refers to S_1 (low) and S_{16} (high) intensities of Grass PS-22 photostimulator.

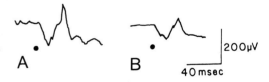

Figure 5.1 Appropriate light adaptation for eliciting photopic ERG responses is easily judged by observing the character of the waveforms. If the background illumination is correct, a normal eye will produce a brisk, fast response, about 200 uV in amplitude (*A*). Excessively bright backgrounds will reduce the photopic ERG (*B*). The examiner should increase the background brightness until a diminution of response to a high intensity occurs and then back off until a normal amplitude once agains appears.

with a "pure" cone response. As the background is raised, a normal cone response is obtained (Fig. 5.1A). Most laboratories report photopic responses to a high intensity flash (typically to an intensity 16 on the Grass PS-22 apparatus) of about 150 to 200 μV with a time-to-peak as measured from the flash onset of 20 to 25 msec. If the background (or ganzfeld bowl illumination) is further increased in strength, the amplitude becomes smaller as a result of cone desensitization, but the latency remains about the same (Fig. 5.1B).

Keeping the above in mind, we need only find the point at which further increases in the background start to produce this diminution in the photopic response. There is a simple check on whether the appropriate background intensity has been achieved. Maintain the flash intensity at the same level, switch the repetition rate to 30/second, and observe the trace. The very fast, very bright flicker guarantees that only cones are responding. The burst of flicker also light adapts the retina while it is on. If the average flicker ERG response is about the same amplitude (within 10%) as the single photopic flash amplitude, it shows that the steady background has adapted the retina to the same level as the flicker burst.

6

Determining the Latency of the ERG

OSCILLOSCOPE RECORDING OF THE ERG: ITS USE IN MEASURING B-WAVE LATENCY

Latency measures of the electroretinogram (ERG) b-wave can only be determined by using an oscilloscope, since the inertial characteristics of pen recorders are too great to record accurately the rise time of the wave-form. Many oscilloscopes have sufficient amplification (at least 100 μV/cm is required) to display the ERG. The time base ("X" or horizontal sweep) of the oscilloscope is typically set at 20 msec/cm. In order to display the complete ERG wave-form, the flash stimulus must follow by about 30 msec the appearance of the trace on the oscilloscope screen. Figure 6.1 shows this sequence.

The clinician observes the screen through an oscilloscope camera. The graticule of the screen is set at a low level so that the centimeter markings are just visible. A typical recording is made as follows.

The camera shutter (set for a 1- or 2-second exposure) is tripped immediately before the flash is to be given. As the clinician observes the screen, the single sweep containing the ERG quickly moves across and exposes the film (Polaroid ASA 3000). Beam intensities are determined by trial and error exposures.

Photographing a burst of flicker on an oscilloscope is a little more complicated. It can easily be done, however, if the scope has a "single shot" sweep setting. A burst of flicker is given as soon as the shutter is opened. The first pulse from the photostimulator will trigger a single sweep, and several ERG responses will be captured on the screen. While photoflash stimulators such as the Grass PS-22 do provide an electrical pulse associated with each flash, they do not produce a preflash pulse to start the trace. This precludes the appearance of any trace prior to the ERG recording and makes it difficult to judge whether the response is starting from a "quiet" base line. Fortunately, there are many inexpensive electronic devices available which can trigger a scope-photostimulator combination. Even more fortunately, commercially available units designed for visual electrodiagnostic testing usually incorporate these useful features.

Table 6.1 shows some typical latency measurements for our clinic and gives some idea of expected values.

Unlike amplitudes, latencies and, more particularly, photopic latencies will not vary much between normal patients—hence, their diagnostic interests. Furthermore, in many degenerative diseases of the retina, there will not be any recordable scotopic ERG responses. The cone system, however, may be preserved in the early stages. Therefore, the ERG latencies that one usually reads about are those of the photopic b-waves.

Table 6.1
Typical Latency Measurements

Flash intensity	Light-adapted b-wave latencies	Dark-adapted b-wave latencies (msec)
High (S_{16})	23–25 msec	45–60 (depending on which peak is measured)
Low (S_1) blue	Not used	65–70
Low (S_1) white	Not used	50–55

FLASH ARTIFACT MARKING FOR OSCILLOSCOPE RECORDINGS

Every ERG recording must have a mark indicating the appearance of the flash. Without such information one cannot measure ERG latencies or confidently dis-

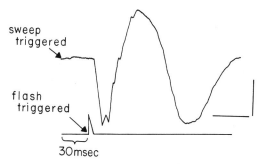

sweep triggered

flash triggered

30msec

Figure 6.1 To measure the latency characteristics of an ERG wave-form on a scope recording, it is essential that a flash artifact appear either on a second trace, as shown, or if it can be made unobtrusive, on the response trace itself. It is useful to have the response trace start about 30 msec ahead of the flash presentation so that a sample of base line precedes the ERG. Calibration: 40 msec and 200 μV.

tinguish the ERG response from a blink or eye movement. In scope recording, a photoartifact from the flash may appear (as a fine spike) right on the ERG trace. Such photoartifacts rarely appear in polygraph recordings because the pens do not respond quickly enough. If such artifacts are not apparent on the scope record, then an oscilloscope with two beams must be used (Fig. 6.1). Most photostimulators like the Grass provide a pulse, the amplitude of which varies with the intensity setting and serves as a flash marker.

GANZFELD STIMULATION

Figure 6.2 shows the theoretical production of ERGs from a retina stimulated directly by a flash lamp. Areas of the retina which receive only small amounts of scattered illumination generate smaller, longer latency b-waves than areas which are more directly stimulated. Since the recorded ERG is a summation of both scattered and directly stimulated portions of the retina, the *average* latency time from

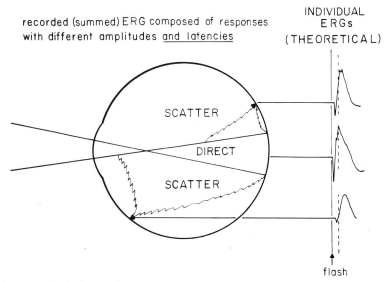

recorded (summed) ERG composed of responses with different amplitudes <u>and latencies</u>

INDIVIDUAL ERGs (THEORETICAL)

SCATTER

DIRECT

SCATTER

flash

Figure 6.2 An open flash directed at the eye produces an intense image on the retina and a great deal of scattered light throughout the interior of the eye. The ERGs produced by the weaker portions of the scattered light would have longer latencies (and smaller amplitudes) than the ERG generated by the directly imaged flash. Since the recorded ERG is a summation of all electrical activity, wave-form latency estimates cannot be accurately determined.

recorded (summed) ERG composed of homogeneous responses because retina is <u>evenly</u> illuminated

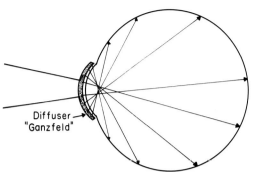

Diffuser—
"Ganzfeld"

Figure 6.3 A ganzfeld bowl or diffuser over the contact lens electrode spreads the incident light flash evenly over the retina. For accurate latency determinations, some form of ganzfeld illumination is required.

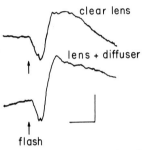

clear lens

lens + diffuser

↑
flash

Figure 6.4 Diffusing the light evenly over the retina produces an enhancement of the ERG response because a great deal more light reaches the retinal periphery. This occurs despite the fact that the diffuser itself absorbs a considerable amount of light. Calibration lines: 40 msec and 200 μV.

this type of recording will be longer, as compared to a b-wave generated from a retina stimulated by the same flash which has its intensity spread uniformly across the entire retina. Figure 6.3 shows how a diffuser in front of the eye produces such homogeneous light distribution. There are many ways to produce such complete field or "ganzfeld" illumination. These include large, matte-white diffuser bowls,[14] indirectly illuminated by a flash lamp, or diffuser shields fitted over the contact lens electrode itself.[15] The latter technique is shown in Figure 6.3. A piece of Ping-Pong ball makes an excellent, inexpensive diffuser. Comparison of an ERG record with and without the diffuser on the lens (Fig. 6.4) shows the amplitude increase when the flash is spread evenly over most of the retina.

Even though the Ping-Pong diffuser reduces the intensity of the flash by about 85%, the response is, if anything, a little larger than the direct flash stimulus. Because the light is spread in such a homogeneous fashion to almost all regions of the retina, even remote peripheral areas contribute to the potential. Thus, a patient with cataractous changes would not be expected to have a particularly attenuated ERG. Indeed, most cataracts, even those dense enough to preclude fundus observation, behave as intraocular ganzfelds, and quite respectable ERG amplitudes may be expected under these circumstances.

7

Separation of Rod and Cone ERG Activity

For purposes of diagnosis it often becomes necessary for the examiner to separate and evaluate rod and cone activity. Intrinsic differences between the two systems, already alluded to in earlier sections, enable us to make the distinction. We have, for example, mentioned the difference in rod and cone spectral sensitivity, their distinct operating characteristics at low and high levels of retinal adaptation, as well as the ability of cones to follow high flicker rates. Many psychophysical functions make use of these (and other) attributes, with the result that a great variety of subjective test procedures, e.g. dark adaptation, acuity vs. luminance, flicker fusion, and brightness discrimination, show a clear "break" indicative of the visual system switching from rod to cone activity. Analogous electrical testing of the retina using the electroretinogram (ERG) may also be performed. With infants and young children, ERG testing may, of course, be the only alternative.

Data from such types of psychophysical studies give us all the information we require to elicit electrical signals from the retina which clearly distinguish rod and cone activity. We will, however, concern ourselves with just those few ERG procedures that are in general use for such purposes.

FLICKER STIMULATION

An intense light flashing on and off at rates exceeding 15 per second will elicit a "following" response of ERG b-wave activity. As shown in Figure 7.1, for every flash there will be a well-defined b-wave—the so-called flicker response. If the patient has no cone function (e.g., the rod monochromat), no flicker response is evident. If the ERG recording system is designed to detect the first response to the flickering light and not just later ones (those referred to as "steady state flicker"), a small initial wavelet will be recorded. This initial response is, of course, produced by the rod system, which cannot respond repetitively because of the high level of light adaptation and, most importantly, because of the fast flicker rate. Thus, while both rods and cones will respond briskly to a single intense flash, the rods "turn off" slowly while the cone membrane potential returns quickly to preflash base line values. In practical terms, this translates into a relatively long refractory period for rods—long enough so that further stimulation in less than 100 msec is not possible. Therefore, flash repetition rates faster than 10/sec simply do not allow rods time to recover. Thus, clear separation between rods and cones on a strictly temporal basis is quite easily achieved. Holding a red filter in front of a 30/sec flash to further ensure "pure" cone response is, in view of the foregoing discussion, superfluous, but useful if one does not wish to dazzle (or grossly light adapt) the patient.

RED FLASH STIMULATION IN THE DARK-ADAPTED EYE

In many circumstances, it is difficult to obtain a good flicker response. Patients with nystagmus or photophobia, or those who are apprehensive, have a particularly hard time relaxing their lids during the brief exposure to an intense flicker stimulus. In such instances, and also as a double check on the photopic flicker, a completely different maneuver is recommended—a deep red flash to the dark-adapted eye. The latter can be obtained by using the red filter supplied by the Grass Instrument Company, or a commercially available broadband gelatin filter like the Kodak Wrattan no. 92. A moderately bright flash setting (S_8 on the Grass stimulator) will result in a double-peaked ERG response, such as the one shown in Figure 7.2.

When the eye is dark adapted, the rod system is obviously dominant. However, even in this state cones can also contribute to an ERG elicited by a flash—of any color. The reason why a red flash works to produce a clear rod and cone separation is a combination of two factors. First, cones are intrinsically a faster system, and we would expect them to respond to any mod-

erately bright flash before the slower acting rods. Second, while rods contribute most of the dark-adapted potential, red light is the least efficient portion of the spectrum for rod excitation. By the time the longer latency rods respond to the flash, the cone ERG is completed. Therefore, the color of the flash and the faster latency of the cones guarantee that the second, slower, large peak reflects activity from the late responding rod photoreceptors.

In practice, we have found that even greater separation of the two systems can be achieved with a dim red flash (S_2 Grass setting) presented every second and summing a dozen or so flashes using a signal averager. The final wave-form after such processing, however, does not vary from that of Figure 7.2 in its appearance. However, the less light presented to the dark-adapted eye, the more reliable the separation attained.

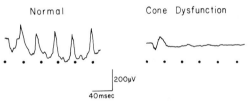

Normal   Cone Dysfunction

200μV

40msec

Figure 7.1 A high intensity flash presented 30 times/second produces, in the normal eye, a following response which indicates that the vast majority of retinal cones are functioning. Patients with diseases affecting the cone system will show a decreased, or absent, flicker response. The initial small ERG seen in such patients represents a single response from the rods, which are unable to recover fast enough to follow flash rates exceeding several per second.

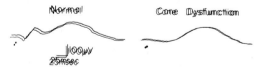

Normal   Cone Dysfunction

100μV

25msec

Figure 7.2 A very quick estimate of retinal cone function can also be obtained by presenting a dim red flash to the dark-adapted eye. Rod and cone systems respond sufficiently differently to the red flash to allow complete separation of the corresponding ERG activity. The first small wavelet derives from the cone system and the later larger one from the rods. Patients with decreased cone function will only show the rod portion of the ERG wave.

BALANCED SCOTOPIC STIMULATION

The clinician will often come across a report in which an investigator, wishing to separate rod and cone activity, uses what is called "balanced scotopic flashes." Unfortunately, the theoretical basis for the procedure is rarely spelled out.

Figure 7.3 shows the scotopic and photopic luminosity curves of the human eye. In the scotopic curve, the peak (λ max) at 500 nm and general shape of the curve indicate that rhodopsin-containing rods are the primary generating elements. The curve allows us to compare the relative (scotopic) sensitivity of the eye with respect to all the wavelengths used. For example, 2 log units more intensity (100 times more) at wavelength 640 nm are required to attain a "just visible" threshold, as compared to one at 440 nm. By changing the experimental conditions, the photopic (cone) luminosity curve can be derived and is shown next to the scotopic curve. Note that the λ_{max} is now shifted from 500 to 560 nm (a shift first observed by Purkinje and named after him). Note that the sensitivity

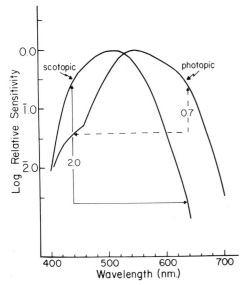

Figure 7.3 Theoretical basis for fabricating a pair of "scotopically balanced" ERG stimuli. The spectral sensitivity characteristics of the rod and cone systems differ so markedly from each other that matching the intensity for a pair of wavelengths requires quite dissimilar neutral filter values. As shown in the figures, there is a 2.0 log unit difference between the 440 and 620 nm pair of wavelengths under scotopic (rod) conditions. Note that the same pair of wavelengths require only a 0.7 log unit intensity adjustment to equate them with respect to luminance when the cone system is operating.

difference between 440 nm and 640 nm is no longer 2.0 but 0.7 log units. Look once again at the scotopic curve. It would have been perfectly possible to "fool" the eye and obtain the same threshold for 440 and 640 nm points by decreasing the intensity of the 440 nm wavelength with a 2 log unit neutral density filter in the light path. With the 2.0 compensating neutral filter in place, those two wavelengths, 440 and 640 nm, are response equivalent—*but only for the rod system*. If experimental conditions were changed to measure cone sensitivity, then the scotopically balanced 440 and 640 nm flashes would *not* elicit equivalent responses. The longer (640 nm) wavelength would appear brighter and the shorter (440 nm) wavelength dimmer than they did for the rods since only 0.7 log units now sep-

arate them. In sum, scotopically balanced pairs of wavelengths yielding equivalent responses for the rod system are clearly *not* equivalent when the cone system is activated. Applying these principles to ERG procedures, we find we have to make similar adjustments.

To set up scotopically balanced ERG stimuli, the following steps are required.

1. Fully dark adapt a *normal* patient.

2. Choose two broad band filters (of the Kodak Wrattan type), one transmitting predominantly red (Wrattan no. 92) and one predominantly blue (Wrattan no. 44A).

3. Keeping the flash lamp at a constant intensity (about S_8 or S_4 on the Grass stimulator), add sufficient neutral density filters to either the blue or red (it will probably be the blue flash) so that the b-wave amplitudes for the red and blue are *exactly the same*. Figure 7.4 (*top*) shows a pair of equal amplitude ERG responses to blue and red flashes in the dark-adapted eye. Thus, for any individual with a normal scotopic system, the examiner would have at hand appropriate filters to generate equal amplitude responses.

The only purpose of constructing a balanced pair of filters that yield equiamplitudes responses in a normal dark-adapted eye is to establish a starting point for partitioning out identifiable responses from *only* the rod and *only* the cone system when we *unbalance* the system. The unbalancing is accomplished in the manner described in step 4 and illustrated in Figure 7.4.

4. What would be the effect on this pair of balanced responses if the retina was now light adapted, say, by a steady background luminance applied to a ganzfeld bowl? To answer the question, one need only recall the difference between rod and cone absolute sensitivity and the difference in their spectral sensitivities. A dim light background will do two things— markedly attenuate the rod responses and allow the photopic system to reveal itself. The light background completely "unbalances" and tends to separate responses from rods and cones. The separation is made even more complete by the use of

blue and red flashes. Note how different in appearance the light-adapted blue and red ERG responses are in Figure 7.4, as compared to those of the dark-adapted pair. The slow, small-amplitude blue response is, in fact, a rod response weakly responding in the presence of the light background. In contrast, the red flash now elicits the fast, brisk response so characteristic of the cone system.

To further dramatize the separation of responses, the background may be raised to higher levels. The blue flash will then elicit *no* ERG response at all, but the red flash response will hardly be changed in appearance. We have now altered the operating characteristic of the retina so that only cone activity can be electrically detected. However, eliminating the blue flash ERG response altogether serves little purpose for diagnosis. What is useful is a light background level such as the one shown in Figure 7.4 which allows *both* systems to manifest themselves.

The application of a pair of balanced scotopic stimuli presented against a background of appropriate brightness becomes obvious when the flashes are given, not to a normal eye, but to one in which rod or cone activity is selectively diminished. In the discussion which follows we shall consider (for the sake of brevity) only the

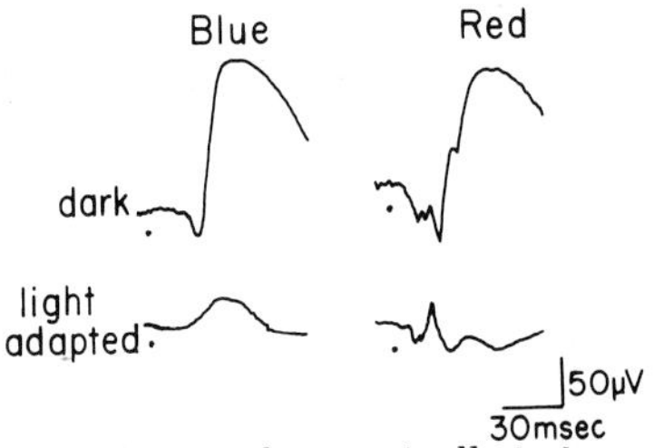

Blue   Red

dark

light adapted

50μV
30msec

Figure 7.4 A pair of scotopically balanced blue and red flashes presented to the dark-adapted eye produces approximately equal amplitude responses. The same pair of stimuli produce responses which differ markedly in appearance if the eye is light adapted. Should the retina have defective cone function, the response to the red flash would be markedly attenuated or absent. By regulating the strength of light adaptation, one can quantify the degree of cone contribution to the ERG response.

responses elicited by the "balanced" red and blue flashes in the presence of a steady light background.

The bottom pair of responses in Figure 4.4 are from a normal eye. However, if the cones of the retina are malfunctioning (e.g., congenital rod monochromatism or a patient with progressive cone dysfunction), the red flash response will be absent. The blue flash, on the other hand, will not differ much from normal. Diseases affecting the rods more than the cones (early retinitis pigmentosa and some forms of congenital nyctalopia) will produce the opposite effect, viz., the blue flash ERG would be smaller than normal while the cone (red flash) ERG is less affected. To what degree rod or cone ERG amplitudes will be diminished will, of course, depend on the type of retinal degeneration and at what stage of the disease the test is performed. Thus, balanced scotopic stimuli can, in ideal cases, provide an almost quantitative estimate of rod and cone malfunction.

In our experience we have found the photopic flicker (30/sec) to be the quickest estimate of retinal cone function; it gives accurate measures of the amplitude and latency of the photopic b-wave. However, there are many situations where one would like to know if the rods as well as the cones are being affected by some generalized retinal disease. There are now so many categories of "cone-rod degeneration," "progressive cone degeneration," and forms of achromatopsia, that it becomes essential to evaluate the rod system as well as the cones. For a quick estimate, we generally use the single low intensity red flash, signal averaged several times if possible. The response to such a stimulus will show in one photograph the relative contribution of the rods and cones to a weak flash. In fact, since very little light can be used to produce the double-humped ERG, the response of the dark-adapted eye to a red flash can be considered (along with the balanced scotopic pair technique) a most sensitive indicator of not just the cone system but of the rods as well.

8

Recording Electrical Activity from the Fovea

Since the clinical electroretinogram (ERG) is a response generated by large areas of retina, it should be clear to the reader that its usefulness in detecting localized pathology is necessarily limited. Despite its virtue as a measure of generalized dysfunction, there are a great number of conditions, namely, those specifically affecting the macular region, which cannot be evaluated by the usual ERG procedures. Several elaborate and sophisticated techniques have been designed to refine the ERG so that small retinal areas may be examined.

The art of obtaining electrical signals from small, preselected areas of the retina has been practiced for almost 20 years.[16] However, only recently have the techniques been simplified sufficiently to consider using them routinely in clinical situations.

Historically, two major obstacles prevented the experimenter from measuring electrical activity that originates in a small (fovea or macula size) region on the retina: signal detection and stray light stimulation. The first difficulty involves the detection of this small ERG signal generated in response to the small patch of stimulated retina. Raising the amplification to increase an ERG signal of only a few microvolts will also increase the background noise. Since the so-called base line on most ERG recordings is itself about 5 to 10 μV in amplitude, if the gain (amplification) is increased 10 times, the base line noise will be similarly augmented with no net enhancement of the ERG signal.

Most of the background noise encountered is random in nature, i.e., not related in any direct way with the response of the eye to light stimuli. The summation or averaging process of the microcomputer-based signal averager takes advantage of the fact that background noise amplitude fluctuations are not synchronized to the onset of the stimulus. The averager starts its analysis sequence on a command which also presents the stimulus to the eye. Only the signal generated by the retina in response to the stimulus occurs at the same time and with the same wave-form characteristics. Random fluctuations, on the other hand, simply tend to sum toward a zero value since at any given time there is just as much change of a positive-going fluctuation as a negative-going one. Only the temporally synchronized ERG signal is enhanced by such averaging. Such signal-to-noise enhancement can usually produce detectable ERG recordings of just a few microvolts. While signal averaging techniques are usually not required for the routine ERG recordings, the capability may prove useful for patients producing low amplitude signals or where fluctuations such as eye movement or eye blinks may mask the ERG. For this reason, and because of the fact that such processing is required for visual evoked potential (VEP) recording, most manufacturers integrate signal averaging capacity into their basic ERG systems.

The second problem, that of dealing with stray light, is a more subtle obstacle. The first ERG researchers attempting such recordings realized that the light intensity within the stimulus area must be kept dim enough so as not to excite photoreceptors outside the area with scattered stray light. Testing for the unwanted activity induced by stray light was done by placing the small stimulus spot on the optic nerve head. If an ERG was elicited, it must have originated from stray light activating elements of the retina outside the nerve head. If no ERG was recorded, even after many signal averagings, it was assurance that the effective stimulus would scatter light at least not larger than the size of the nerve head.[16]

It is also possible to reduce stray light effects by desensitizing a large portion of the retina with a steady light and then superimposing a flashing stimulus light within the area. The underlying assumption here is that any stray light from the stimulus will not be able to photoactivate surrounding retina which is already being desensitized by light backgrounds, the intensity of which is greater than any induced effect of scatter from the stimulus. The response may be further enhanced if consideration is given to the spectral sensitivity of the rod-dominated areas surrounding the fovea. Aiba et al.,[17] for example, used a large blue-green steady background and superimposed a small flickering spot of deep red light to obtain foveal ERGs.

However, the sorts of optical equipment and patient control required to obtain foveal ERGs under such circumstances were not easily accessible to the clinician. Some years ago Riggs and his students[18] devised a technique for controlling stray light that was based on a completely different (and ingenious) principle. They optically generated a pattern of bars which appeared to move back and forth. The alternating shift was just one bar width long so that black stripes seemed to be replaced with light stripes and vice versa. Because no net change in luminance was produced by the movement, any light falling on nondirectly stimulated areas of retina appeared to be steady. In other words, only that portion of the retina underlying the image of alternating light and dark bars produced the ERG. In practice, care must be taken to make sure that the average luminance across the whole pattern remains constant. For example, the same number of dark bars must be replaced with white ones. If a properly calibrated pattern is projected onto a diffusing screen, which effectively destroys the intensity variations in the image, only an even illumination is seen. This occurs despite the fact that the bars of light and dark in the original pattern are reversing back and forth. Such a demonstration shows that stray light from the pattern is "seen" by the retina as a steady light. Since the ERG is a transient response, it can only be generated by changing light intensity. The only areas of the retina receiving changing light fluxes are those underlying the shifting pattern on bars. Technically speaking, we are summating local ERGs from small retinal regions which are being alternately thrust into darkness and light as the dark bars suddenly change to light ones.

Armington[19] has used this technique to demonstrate the linear summative properties of the retina. His data also provide practical areal limitations. One would like to know, for example, how small an area can be stimulated with the expectation of a detectable response, for the macula is a rather large area, and even the fovea, usually taken to be 5° in diameter, is still gross compared to the tiny foveola, the integrity of which is required for "20/20" acuity. Armington's data indicate that a signal can be reliably recorded from a square area no smaller than 3° across.

If a Burian-Allen-type contact lens electrode is used for recording the foveal ERG, one can be certain that the retinal image will be degraded and the game lost before the start button is pressed. Ideally, the cornea should not be obscured at all, and for optical reasons neither should the pupil be maximally dilated nor the accommodation be paralyzed with a cycloplegic—unless compensated for by the appropriate lenses. A foil electrode,[20] or some variation of it,[21] where the electrode hooks over the lid must be used so that the natural viewing optics of the eye are preserved.

One final, technical point must be mentioned. Eye blinks and slight eye movements, which are annoying enough artifacts in ordinary ERG recording, are catastrophic when attempting to detect local ERGs. To overcome the latter problem, one must have available an artifact rejection function associated with the signal averager. This feature is usually built into the higher quality averagers and designated as a "pre-analysis buffer" or "artifact reject." The averager with this option "looks" at the signal before it is analyzed and, depending on the setting chosen, rejects voltage fluctuations much greater than the size of local ERG signals. The pattern ERG therefore can be expected to record a gross potential from the foveal area, but one cannot expect this potential to be rigorously correlated with small amounts of visual loss. The one exception to this observation relates to recent findings in amblyopia,[22, 23] in which patterns subtending several degrees in size show dramatic ERG reduction compared to those in fellow normal eyes. However, most amblyopes have also been shown to have reduced contrast sensitivity functions over a wide range of spatial frequencies.[24] This particular visual abnormality may involve loss of retinal function over an area far exceeding that of the foveola. However, for visual loss due to causes other than amblyopia, the VEP is probably a better estimate of subjective acuity.[25]

9

Electrooculography

The normal eyeball acts like a battery with a measurable voltage between the cornea and the back of the globe. The current flow is oriented so that the cornea is "voltage-positive" relative to the posterior pole. This is sometimes referred to as the standing (or resting) potential of the eye.

If electrodes are placed on either side of the eye and the globe is rotated, a difference can be recorded between the electrodes. If the electrodes are connected to a polygraph, the voltage changes are translated into pen movement: as the eye moves to the left, the pen will move up; right eye movements produce a downward pen swing. Thus, eye movement is translated into an electrical change—the electrooculogram (EOG).

If the eye executes saccades between two fixed points, it is reasonable to assume that the EOG will have a constant amplitude corresponding to the left and right eye-swings. In fact, the EOG undergoes small cyclic variations in amplitude because the current flow of the globe slowly waxes and wanes. It has also been observed that EOG amplitudes change markedly if the eye is left in darkness for some minutes and then exposed to a bright steady light.

Figure 9.1 shows how the EOG changes in the dark and light phases. Each *black circle* on the figure represents several right- or left-averaged EOG responses. The lowest value reached while the eyes track saccades in the dark is called the "dark trough." The peak amplitude achieved against a steady light background is called the "light peak." The light peak/dark trough ratio (or "light rise") is measured in millimeters of pen swing or oscilloscope scale divisions and is an index (the Arden index) of retinal function.[26] A ratio value of 1.80 (180%) is considered the lower limit of normal—although, like the ERG, index values are age dependent.[27] Usually, 5 minutes of preadaptation at room light levels are required to establish steady EOG base line values. Fifteen minutes of darkness followed by 15 minutes of light adaptation are the typical retinal adaptation conditions used for this test. The patient, of course, does not have to continually execute saccades; he need only make several each minute during the recording period.

Most EOG recordings require that the patient alternately fixate two points about 1 meter apart. The points are usually small flashing lights located on either side of a large illuminated screen, the patient-screen distance being about 1 meter. Since many patients find it difficult to perform smooth, accurate saccades between the two alternating flashes of light, in our own laboratory we have facilitated the EOG recording for both patient and clinician in the following way. Rather than using two isolated fixation points, a black strip of plastic containing about 30 light-emitting diodes (LEDs) is directly mounted on a commercially available 24 x 36 inch self-illuminated drawing board. Figure 9.2 shows the strip and board. The LEDs are sinusoidally spaced along the length of the strip so that when they are sequentially pulsed, they appear to the eye as a bright spot of red light moving back and forth in a pendular motion. The board contains four (40-watt) fluorescent lamps which produce the high levels of light adaptation required to elicit a maximum light rise. The patient simply follows the point of light as it sweeps across the strip at about twice/second. The recording polygraph speed or oscilloscope sweep is adjusted to 5 mm/sec so that the accuracy of the eye movements can be checked (see Fig. 9.3).

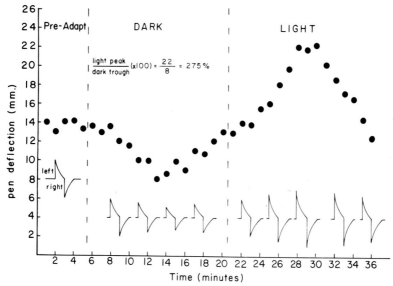

Figure 9.1 Graphical representation of light-induced changes in the EOG. Electrical responses produced by fixed saccadic movements are sampled in the dark and during a period of intense light adaptation. The *black circles* represent the average pen swing amplitude (in millimeters) of several saccades taken during the 5-minute preadaptation period, 15 minutes of darkness, and 15 minutes in the presence of background light. *Insets* show how the individual EOG responses decrease in the dark and increase in the light. The greatest EOG amplitude achieved in the light (*light peak*) is divided by the lowest amplitude in the dark (*dark trough*) and the calculated ratio is expressed as a percent.

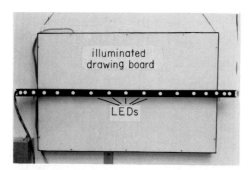

Figure 9.2 Apparatus for producing light-induced EOG responses. A black plastic bar containing about 20 LEDs is mounted across a 4-tube fluorescent drawing box. The LEDs (represented by *white circles*) are distributed in sinusoidal fashion across the bar (closer together on the ends and farther apart in the center) and are pulsed sequentially. The LEDs appear to execute a harmonic (pendulum) motion as they are activated from one end of the bar to the other. For patients who have difficulty in executing saccades between two distant fixation points, this technique ensures accurate tracking movements. Sample tracings with the apparatus are shown in Figure 9.3.

If the paper speed or scope sweep is stepped down to a very slow speed (0.25 mm/sec), the saccades run together, and several of them form a thick rectangular block. This maneuver creates a response averaging of sorts which eliminates the tedious measuring of individual saccades during the recording period. In Figure 9.3, the polygraph paper drive motor is stopped between recordings so that individual minutes can be discerned. As the figure shows, a complete 45-minute recording, with the light rise clearly seen, is immediately available at the conclusion of the session.

PATIENT PREPARATION AND RECORDING CONDITIONS FOR THE EOG

Silver-silver chloride or gold disc electrodes (8 mm) are fixed to the medial and lateral canthi of each eye using a procedure similar to that described for the electroretinogram (ERG) reference electrode. The patient may wear his distance spectables after the electrodes are affixed if needed for sharper vision. A ground clip electrode makes contact on the ear with a bit of electrode jelly. A typical electrode placement is shown in Figure 9.4.

The 5-minute base line recording (Fig. 9.3) serves the purpose of acquainting the patient with his task and enables the cli-

nician to see how well the saccades are performed. At this time, the amplitude of the polygraph pen swing or oscilloscope trace should be adjusted to compensate for the expected increase during light adaptation. For example, if a polygraph pen has a maximum excursion of 3 cm it is adjusted during the preadaptation period so that the amplitudes do not exceed 1.5 cm. In the dark they may go to half this value (0.75

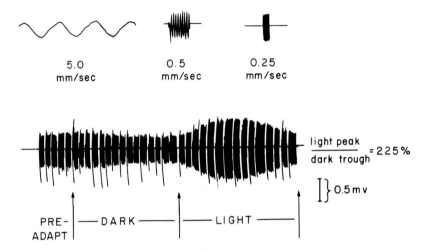

Figure 9.3 If the eye follows a moving light executing harmonic motion (see Fig. 9.2), the polygraph record will have sinusoidal appearance (5.0 mm/sec trace). Very slow recording speeds compress the individual recordings together, allowing the clinician to quickly measure the resulting solid block. This technique also produces a complete representation of the dark- and light-induced changes on a small length of paper as shown, without the necessity for tedious measuring and graphing.

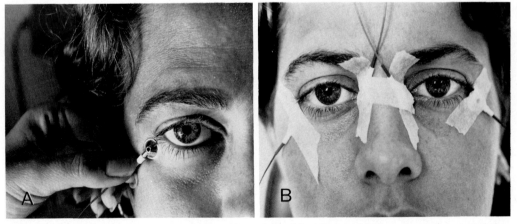

Figure 9.4 Preparation for EOG testing. Silver-silver chloride or gold disc electrodes containing a dab of conducting jelly are affixed close to the nasal and temporal canthi of each eye. The areas have been cleaned with alcohol and rubbed dry prior to electrode attachment.

cm), and even if the light rise is as high as 300%, the pen swing will only reach 2.25 cm at the peak.

The reader may find a word on the light adaptation requirements appropriate. While actual photometric values given by Arden and Kelsey[28] are said to be optimal at about 2000 trolands, there is a rule of thumb which can simplify matters for the clinician. One has only to be assured that the background luminance is high enough to obtain a light rise of about 250% in a group of young normals. We have found that even pupil dilatation does not change the Arden ratio by more than 10%, a point that is useful for working with patients who are photophobic. The angular extent of the light-adapted field also plays a role in the magnitude of the light rise. Fishman and his coworkers[29] have determined that fields subtending an angle smaller than 30° at the eye produce erroneous Arden ratios. If the EOG is performed in the confines of a ganzfeld bowl provided with a sufficiently high level of background illumination, the latter problem is simply dealt with. The light box arrangement, suggested above, provides a rectangle subtending about 60 x 40 degrees when the patient is placed 1 meter in front of it.

ORIGIN OF THE EOG POTENTIALS

It is important to distinguish between the standing (or resting) potential of the eye (RPE) and the *light-induced changes* in the standing potential. The latter effect is, of course, what we mean when we refer to an "EOG" recording. To understand the clinical implications of the EOG light rise, two factors must be clearly understood: (1) the light rise is *generated* by light stimulation of the photoreceptor-RPE complex, and (2) the light rise is *detected* only if certain structures in the midretinal layer are normal. Some explanation of these statements is required.

Quantal absorption by photoreceptors initiates a decrease in K^+ concentration which in turn hyperpolarizes the pigment epithelial cells.[30] The hyperpolarization can be seen in DC recordings of the ERG as the c-wave and late-appearing light peak.[31] Under the influence of a steady light background, pigment epithelial hyperpolarization increases, reaching a peak in several minutes, and then decreases to base line values. The EOG as we record it is probably a reflection of the large light peak amplitude changes.[32] It is important to note that since direct measure of the very slow light changes is quite difficult to determine, the EOG may provide some measure of pigment epithelium integrity. However, the light rise (or the c-wave) cannot be detected without the presence of functioning rods. Therefore, it is fair to say that the light rise of the EOG is a measure of the receptor-pigment epithelium complex.

However, two clinical examples demonstrate that the EOG light rise is absent while the RPE-photoreceptor complex is normal. In one form of congenital stationary nightblindness, no ERG b-wave is detectable, but a normal EOG light rise is generated.[33] Also, central retinal artery occlusion obliterates both the EOG light rise and ERG b-wave but does not interfere with photoreceptor function.[5] In these examples the midretinal cells necessary for the detection of the EOG light rise are compromised, producing an abnormal Arden ratio. Thus, the EOG light rise *reflects* activity from the midretinal layers, such activity being *initiated* by the stimulated pigment epithelial cells.

10

Visual Evoked Cortical Potentials

Since the clinical electroretinogram (ERG) and electrooculogram (EOG) are responses generated by large areas of retina, it should be clear to the reader that their usefulness in detecting localized pathology is necessarily limited. Despite their virtue as a measure of generalized dysfunction, there are a number of conditions, namely, those specifically affecting the macular region, which cannot be evaluated by these procedures. The sophisticated technique whereby the ERG can be recorded from the fovea has been described in Chapter 8. In this chapter, we discuss a technique for evaluating foveal activity which is considerably simpler to perform than the local ERG—the visual evoked cortical potential (VEP). The instrumentation is identical to that already described in Chapter 9. While the VEP affords an accurate assessment of foveal function, the clinician should keep in mind that the potentials recorded are, in effect, only *indirect* measures of the fovea. These potentials, generated in the occipital cortex, represent the end stages of visual processing elicited by appropriate stimulation of the retina. In spite of this limitation, the VEP can provide excellent correlative measures of many subtle aspects of foveal function.

RECORDING THE VEP

The foveal areas are generously represented in the occipital cortex, and are anatomically located on a superficial aspect of area 17 which makes them accessible to examination by scalp electrodes. In fact, a disc electrode placed about 1 cm above the inion will detect potentials that predominantly reflect foveal activity. Figure 10.1 illustrates the technique of electrode placement for VEP recording. Since VEP amplitudes as detected by the remotely placed scalp electrode are extremely small, a signal averager of the type described for recording foveal ERGs must be employed. For specifics, the reader should consult the review article by Sokol.[34]

While the VEP is hardly a new test, it is only with the development of appropriate stimulus generators and electronic averaging devices that VEP recording can be performed with the same ease of operation and confidence as the ERG. The most commonly used stimulus in the past was a light flash which diffusely illuminated the retina in the same manner as in the standard ERG recording. While the responses produced by diffuse flash stimulation show marked interindividual variability in wave-form and amplitude, this approach can still be useful as an assessment of gross foveal function in infants and young children, in the presence of opaque media, as a rapid comparison of visual function between a normal and abnormal eye, and as a test for malingering in a patient who claims severe (<20/400) visual loss.

However, in most cases, when the above are not a consideration, the stimulus now widely used for eliciting maximal cortical activity is an electronically generated checkerboard pattern displayed on the screen of a TV monitor.[35] The checkerboard squares reverse from black to white and back at a selected alternation rate, but the screen maintains a constant average luminance on the retina. In other words, the fovea is detecting the presence of the pattern, not a change in luminance. This type of stimulus also guarantees that areas remote from the fovea do not contribute to

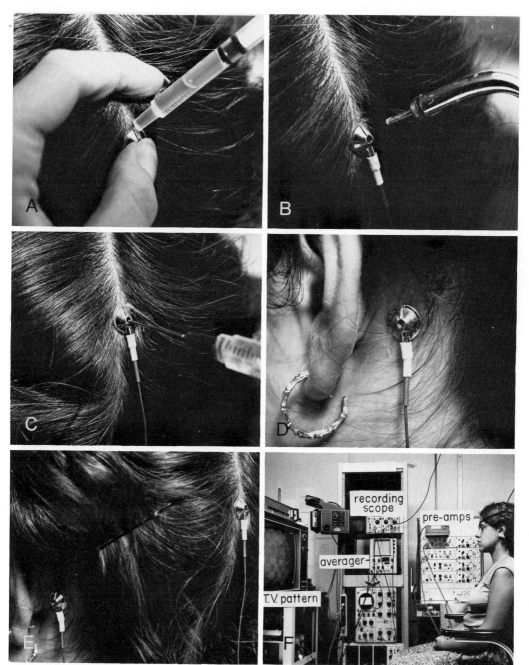

Figure 10.1 Patient preparation for recording the visual evoked potential (VEP). Active electrode placement is most often placed about 1 cm above the inion. The scalp at this position is thoroughly cleaned with alcohol and roughened with the side of a large hypodermic needle or emery cloth. The hair is pushed aside, and the edges of a cupped disc electrode are fixed to the scalp with colloidin (A). A compressed air spray is used to dry the electrode in place (B). Using a blunted hypodermic needle, conducting gel is injected into the cup disc through its top opening (C). An inactive (reference) electrode is fixed over the mastoid bone behind the ear in a manner similar to that of the active electrode (D and E). The resistance between the two electrodes should be about 10 Kohms or less. A ground clip electrode is placed on an ear, and the subject is located in front of the apparatus (F). Typically, the electrode leads are connected to a high gain preamplifier and then to a signal averager. The electronic pattern generator also synchronously drives the averager. The averaged wave-form is either photographed on the averager itself or transferred to an independently operated oscilloscope as shown in F, or written out on an X–Y plotter.

the response since scattered light from the checkerboard as it is imaged on the fovea is seen as a steady background.

CLINICAL APPLICATIONS OF THE VEP

Since cells in the visual cortex are designed to respond most efficiently to complex (textured) patterns of light and less dramatically to diffuse flashes, it follows that greater success in VEP testing will accompany the use of sophisticated photic stimuli such as the reversing checkerboard. Of equal importance is the fact that one can, by manipulating appropriate features in the stimulus pattern, obtain objective correlates of visual acuity, color vision, and contrast sensitivity. In other words, VEP recordings performed in conjunction with meaningful stimuli can give the clinician some idea of what the retina

tells the brain, and what the brain tells "us."

Changing the size of the squares in the checkerboard allows us to objectively determine the smallest check size which produces a VEP. The results of such a procedure would then provide a correlate of visual acuity. Figure 10.2 shows how a stepwise reduction in check size decreases the VEP amplitude.

In some instances it is of benefit to change not check size but just the contrast of a moderate (30 minutes or arc)-sized check. Loss of contrast sensitivity for such large stimuli have been noted in a wide variety of ocular diseases, including macular degeneration,[36] cataract,[37] and optic neuritis.[38] Figure 10.3 shows how decreasing contrast produces marked decrements in the VEP amplitude. The abnormal left eye not only shows smaller amplitudes than the normal fellow eye but also

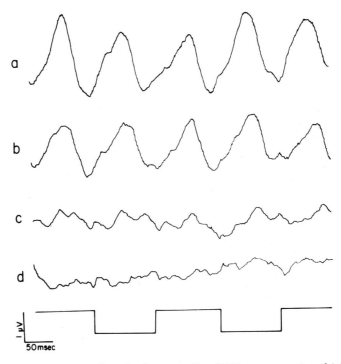

Figure 10.2 Approximating visual acuity by recording VEP responses to a high contrast (60%), reversing checkerboard pattern (alternation rate 10/sec). As the check size is successively decreased from 1° (shown in *trace a*) to 30′ (*b*), 15′ (*c*), 7.5′ (*d*), and 3.8′ (*e*), the responses diminish in amplitude.

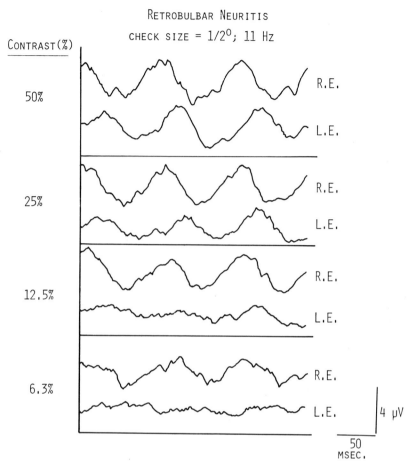

RETROBULBAR NEURITIS

CHECK SIZE = $1/2^O$; 11 Hz

CONTRAST(%)

50%

R.E.
L.E.

25%

R.E.
L.E.

12.5%

R.E.
L.E.

6.3%

R.E.
L.E.

4 µV

50
MSEC.

Figure 10.3 A sensitive indicator of many ocular diseases is the change in VEP response to patterns of diminishing contrast. In the *above traces*, the VEP from the left eye in a patient with a left-sided retrobulbar neuritis shows marked amplitude decreases compared to that of the right eye. At a contrast setting of 25%, the right eye VEP is no different than the response to a pattern with 50% contrast, but the affected left eye has a VEP amplitude that is almost reduced by a factor of two. At 12.5% the right eye is still producing large VEPs while the response to left eye stimulation is extinguished.

changes in the "latency" of the response. Such latency measurements are important in evaluating VEP recordings, especially in suspected cases of optic neuritis. This abnormality of contrast sensitivity is even more meaningful when one considers that the visual acuity of the affected eye is 20/20.

Since it is possible to record foveal ERGs and the VEP with a checkerboard reversal pattern, it is feasible to obtain both types of activity simultaneously. It is of interest, under these circumstances, to contrast the differences between the two responses with regard to detecting foveal disturbance. Figure 10.4 demonstrates such a comparison. Note that when the peripheral portion of the checkerboard is eliminated, the foveal ERG is reduced, relative to the amount of area that was eliminated, while the VEP is hardly changed in amplitude. If the center of the stimulus is removed, the ERG is once again slightly diminished because of areal considerations, while the

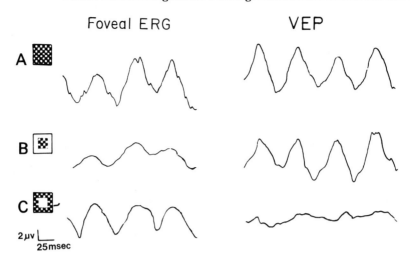

Figure 10.4 Local ERG and VEP activity recorded simultaneously in response to alternating checkerboard stimulus (*A*). Note that when the periphery of the checkerboard is removed (eliminating 75% of the total pattern area), the ERG is diminished proportionately but the VEP amplitude is virtually unchanged (*B*). When just the pattern center is blanked out (representing a loss of 25% of the total area), the ERG is decreased slightly but the VEP is extinguished (*C*). The comparison shows that most of the VEP is derived from a small area of the central fovea whereas the local ERG is a summated response, the amplitude of which is related only to the amount of retina activated.

VEP is practically extinguished. The comparison once again points up the usefulness and sensitivity of the VEP for estimating foveal integrity.

Simultaneous recording of local ERG and VEP is thus possible in a single session and allows evaluation of retinal and cortical aspects of foveal function. Such combined recordings, though technically feasible, are not routinely done in many institutions, but will clearly play a more prominent role in the future.

Section Two

Clinical Section

DIAGNOSTIC GUIDES

Clinical material may be approached in two ways. One can work from the test results back to the disease or, alternatively, list all the well-known disease categories along with their functional findings. This presentation makes use of both approaches. Since the emphasis of this book is on electrodiagnostic techniques and since the clinical test which is most widely available is the electroretinogram (ERG), this section will begin with a brief survey of abnormal ERG findings, presented in the form of "Diagnostic Guides."

Four diagnostic guides (labeled DG-1 through DG-4) illustrating the four main types of abnormal ERG responses are presented in this section. Diseases typically associated with each of four response categories are briefly presented, along with results of electrooculogram (EOG) and subjective retinal testing. Once a disease is identified in one of the guides, its specific characteristics may be more fully explored in succeeding sections of the book, which are organized according to disease categories.

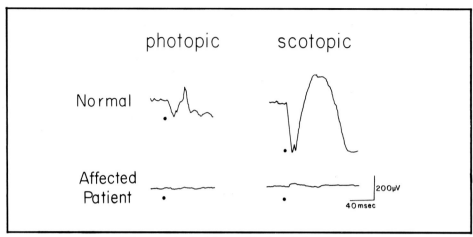

Diagnostic Guide 1   Extinguished ERG.

The ERG shows no detectable response in the light- or dark-adapted retina. The prototype disease producing such a response is retinitis pigmentosa, but several other conditions which also yield extinguished ERGs are listed below. The EOG shows no light rise in the eye which has an extinguished ERG, and dark adaptometry shows elevated cone and rod thresholds.

DG-1
Conditions Associated with an Extinguished ERG

Disease	Retinal sensitivity	Comments
Retinitis pigmentosa (RP) and allied diseases	Elevated rod and cone thresholds	Fundus appearance often diagnostic but can be variable.
Ophthalmic artery occlusion	Elevated rod and cone thresholds	1. Unilateral 2. History of trauma (e.g., anesthesia face mask pressure) 3. In acute stages resembles central retinal artery occlusion
Unilateral retinitis pigmentosa	Elevated rod and cone thresholds (in affected eye)	1. Unilateral 2. Fellow eye completely normal 3. No family history
Chorioretinitis	Thresholds normal in normal-appearing retinal areas	1. If diffuse, may not be distinguishable from RP 2. Serologic tests may help
Metallosis	Elevated rod and cone thresholds	1. Unilateral 2. History 3. Fundus findings and/or ultrasound
Retinal detachment	Elevated rod and cone thresholds	1. Unilateral 2. History 3. Fundus findings and/or ultrasound
Drugs a. 4-Amino quinolines (e.g., chloroquine)	Thresholds variable normal in unaffected retina; elevated in affected areas	History of drug ingestion
b. Phenothiazines	Elevated rod and cone thresholds	Fundus appearance

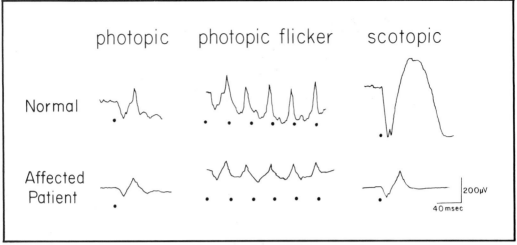

Diagnostic Guide 2   Reduced ERG a- and b-waves.

Reduced ERG a- and b-waves are associated with a variety of ocular disorders. Infrequently, such responses are recorded in progressive forms of primary pigmentary retinopathy. Most commonly, however, attenuated ERGs are found in certain of the stationary varieties of nightblindness, as a result of drug toxicity, and in those diseases which limit the amount of light reaching the retina or in which the pathology is localized to discrete retinal areas.

In the two disease categories where nightblindness may be the presenting or primary symptom, additional tests of visual function may be necessary to arrive at a correct diagnosis. In the primary retinal degenerations, the fundus abnormalities, the visual field changes, and the increased b-wave latencies are distinguishing features. The forms of congenital stationary nightblindness with reduced ERGs, on the other hand, have normal visual fields and normal b-wave latencies. The very slow recovery of adaptation in electrical activity noted for fundus albipunctatus sounds a cautionary note; patients with whitish punctate lesions should always be given the benefit of prolonged dark adaptation, since standard periods of dark adaptation will produce only the very reduced responses shown above.

With regard to those acquired retinal disorders (the last four categories), the degree to which adaptometric findings and electrical potentials are reduced depends on the extent of involved retinal tissue. For drug-induced retinopathy the diminution of function often relates to dosage history. In the case of retinal detachment and chorioretinitis, the ERG amplitudes relate simply to remaining areas of functioning retina. When hemorrhage overlies the retina, the detection of electrical changes depends primarily on how much of the incident light reaches the photoreceptors.

DG-2
Reduced ERG a- and b-waves

Disease	Retinal sensitivity	Comments
Some forms of retinitis pigmentosa and allied diseases	Variable elevation of cone and rod thresholds	1. Fundus abnormalities 2. Visual field abnormalities 3. Decreased EOG light rise 4. b-wave latency may be increased
Congenital stationary night-blindness (CSNB) normal fundus (Type I)	Normal cone thresholds; rod portion of adaptation curve absent	1. Normal visual fields 2. Absent EOG light rise 3. Normal b-wave latency
fundus albipunctatus	Cone and rod systems require extended adaptation to reach normal thresholds	EOG and ERG responses require about 3 hours dark adaptation to reach normal amplitudes
Drugs phenothiazines	Variable loss of cone-rod sensitivity	1. Fundus abnormalities 2. Normal or slightly reduced EOG light rise 3. History of drug ingestion
Retinal detachment	Variable elevation of rod-cone thresholds	1. Variable reduction of EOG light rise 2. Ultrasound confirmation
Vitreous hemorrhage	Usually cannot be performed	"Bright-flash ERG" useful
Chorioretinitis	Normal when tested in normal appearing areas	1. EOG light rise variable 2. ERG b-wave latency normal even when amplitude is decreased

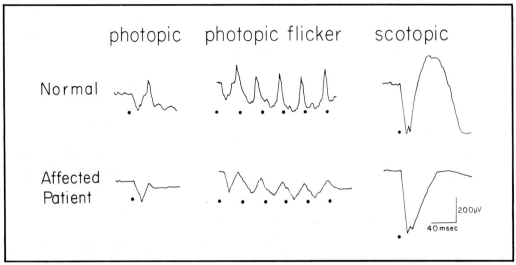

Diagnostic Guide 3   Normal ERG a-wave and reduced b-wave.

The ERG is characterized by a deep a-wave and absent b-wave. The a-wave in most instances will appear deeper than normal. This absence of the b-wave and enhancement of the a-wave is most clearly seen in the three forms of congenital stationary nightblindness. Within this group, an interesting feature of the cone portion of the dark adaptation curve distinguishes Oguchi's disease from fundus albipunctatus (DG-2). Patients with Oguchi's disease attain normal cone thresholds in several minutes, and the cone plateau is extended at this normal level for a prolonged period until the rod-cone break occurs and the slowly descending rod portion appears. In fundus albipunctatus, *both* cone and rod portions require very long periods of time to attain normal sensitivities (compare the adaptation curves in Figs. 14.3 and 14.4).

In juvenile retinoschisis, this ERG abnormality is a distinguishing feature in virtually all cases. The ERG is extremely important in those males who present with cystoid macular changes without the more pathognomic peripheral retinoschisis. Both optic atrophy and central retinal artery occlusion can show an abnormality of the b-wave if there is transsynaptic degeneration involving the bipolar cell region.

The EOG light rise is normal for all the diseases listed in the accompanying table.

DG-3
Conditions Associated with a Normal ERG a-wave and Reduced b-wave

Disease	Retinal sensitivity	Comments
Congenital stationary nightblindness (CSNB) normal fundus (Type II)	Normal cone thresholds; no rod portion of dark adaptation curve	(Compare with similar variety of CSNB in Table DG-2)
Oguchi's disease	Extended dark adaptation curve; thresholds normal after several hours	b-wave will occasionally reach normal levels after a prolonged stay in dark. Metallic reflex in light-adapted eye disappears after a few hours in dark (Mizuo's phenomenon)
with myopia and nystagmus	Normal cone thresholds; no rod branch	
Juvenile retinoschisis	Normal where fundus appears normal	1. Macular cystoid changes may occur without peripheral retinoschisis. 2. Sex-linked transmission
Optic atrophy	Variable; dependent on where retinal area test stimulus is located	Extent of b-wave reduction related to degree of transsynaptic degeneration (ganglion cells to bipolar cell layer)
Central retinal artery occlusion	Variable, threshold levels depend on extent of residual scotoma	1. ERG may be normal in acute stage 2. Extent of b-wave reduction related to degree of transsynaptic degeneration 3. Fellow eye unaffected

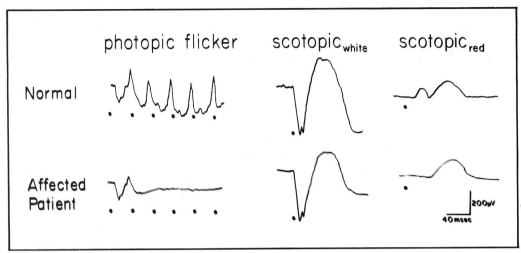

Diagnostic Guide 4 Abnormal photopic and normal scotopic ERG.

Few diseases can be detected with ERG as easily as the generalized cone dysfunctions. Basically, all one needs for diagnosis is the demonstration of an absent photopic flicker response and a normal scotopic ERG response. Some patients exhibit an incomplete form of rod monochromatism, but despite slightly better acuity, crude color sense, and some remnant of retinal cone function, the ERG results are in no way different from the complete form. Patients with progressive cone degeneration may begin life with normal photopic function, and subjective signs and symptoms vary greatly between patients, depending on the stage and severity of the disease. Rod function is preserved throughout the course of the disease. The EOG light rise, being almost entirely dependent on rod function, is normal for both stationary and progressive forms of cone dysfunction.

In addition to the usual ERG light stimuli, a red flash presented to the dark-adapted eye of these patients clearly demonstrates, in one record, the absence of the early cone wavelet and the existence of the slower, later wave, reflecting normal rod activity.

DG-4
Abnormal Photopic, Normal Scotopic ERG

Disease	Retinal sensitivity	Comments
Rod monochromatism	Single-branched dark adaptation curve. No cone-rod break. Rod final thresholds attain normal levels	Variable degree of pigment granularity in macula region. Poor acuity, lack of color vision, photosensitivity, and nystagmus present from birth.
Progressive cone dystrophy	Decreased cone sensitivity dependent on stage of disease. Normal rod function throughout course of disease.	Fundus changes are variable dependent on stage of disease. Nystagmus rarely seen.

11

Generalized Heredo-Degenerations of the Retina

RETINITIS PIGMENTOSA

Retinitis pigmentosa may be considered the prototype of the generalized heredoretinal degenerations. The name itself indicates a rather specific disorder and, in most instances, the manifestations are so typical that the disease is easily recognized and diagnosed. However, it is the closely allied variants of retinitis pigmentosa that may present diagnostic difficulties, and these will be considered in some detail.

In the most common forms of retinitis pigmentosa there is usually a history of poor night vision from childhood, with a later onset of peripheral visual field loss. Most patients have good visual acuity for many years, although in later stages, central vision may also be affected.

The fundus picture (Fig. 11.1) in typical retinitis pigmentosa demonstrates a normal or somewhat pale disc. There is no indication of optic atrophy since histologic studies have shown no degenerative changes in the nerve; any pallor is most likely due to either attenuated vessels on the nerve head with resultant loss of the normal orange-red color or gliosis overlying the nerve. The arterioles show varying degrees of narrowing, and the veins are normal. While the macular area is often spared in the typical case, a wide variety of macular abnormalities have also been described.[39] These include a tapetal-like reflex indicative of pigment epithelial change, a generalized mottling and granularity, or frank pigment epithelial atrophy. In a recent study, cystoid changes in the macula were noted to be present in 70% of patients with retinitis pigmentosa.[40] The fluorescein angiogram in such cases may occasionally show leakage in this area (Fig. 11.2), but usually there is no accumulation of dye. Most of the retina will usually show a somewhat moth-eaten appearance with a variable amount of pigment granularity. The most obvious fundus finding is that of "bone corpuscule" pigmentary clumping which usually begins in the midperiphery and often follows a perivascular distribution. With progression of the disease, there may be increased fallout of the pigment epithelium so that the choroidal pattern becomes clearly visible. Fluorescein angiography in the early stages of the disease shows a normal choriocapillaris pattern (Fig. 11.3). In the late stages there may be some choriocapillaris loss in an irregular, disseminated fashion, often occurring in regions corresponding to the abnormal accumulation of pigment.[41] Patients with retinitis pigmentosa may also show fibrillar vitreal changes and posterior subcapsular cataracts.

It is important to determine any ancillary somatic problems, most particularly impaired hearing. Retinitis pigmentosa occurring together with impaired hearing (Usher's syndrome) has been found in a varying percentage of patients with the autosomal recessive form of retinitis pigmentosa, with estimates ranging from 10 to 70%. The association has also been reported in several families with autosomal dominant mode of transmission.[42] The hearing loss, when present, is usually congenital and can occasionally be combined with mutism. Several longitudinal studies have shown the deafness to be nonprogressive.[43] While retinitis pigmentosa may be associated with deafness, loss of hearing is also found in a variety of other syndromes.[44]

In each case of retinitis pigmentosa, a

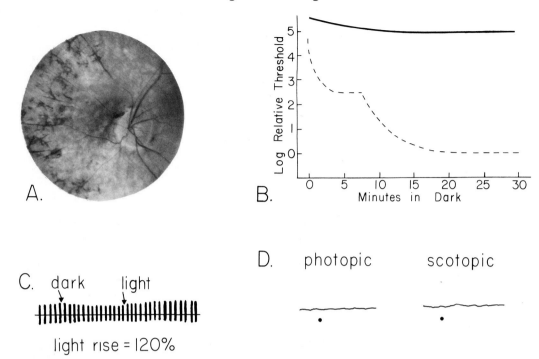

Figure 11.1   Retinitis pigmentosa. *A*, fundus photograph of a 21-year-old female with a history of poor night vision since childhood and poor side vision for 6 years. Visual acuity 20/30 OD and OS. The retina shows a generalized loss of the pigment epithelium with a multitude of strands and spicules of pigment throughout the retinal midperiphery. The arterioles are narrowed, but the optic nerve is normal. There is relative sparing of the macular areas. *B*, dark adaptation. A normal dark adaptation curve showing the cone and rod portion is indicated by the *dash line*. The patient's cone and rod thresholds are markedly elevated (*solid line*). *C*, EOG. The EOG light rise is minimal, and probably represents only base line fluctuations. Normal light rise is at least 175%. *D*, ERG. There is no recordable response under either photopic or scotopic recording conditions.

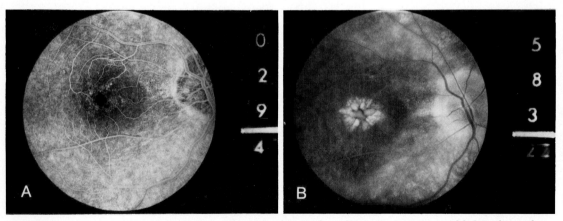

Figure 11.2   Retinitis pigmentosa with cystoid macular changes. A 34-year-old female with longstanding retinitis pigmentosa noted the onset of decreased central vision 4 months prior to being seen. Best corrected visual acuity 20/70 OD and 20/80 OS. Fundus had findings typical of retinitis pigmentosa and also showed macular cystoid changes. *A*, fluorescein angiogram in midvenous phase shows dilated capillaries around the capillary-free zone. *B*, late stage angiogram showing the flower-petal appearance of cystoid macular edema.

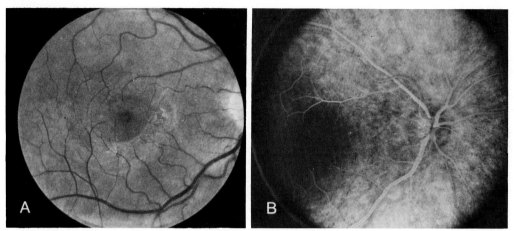

Figure 11.3 Retinitis pigmentosa sine pigmento. A 14-year-old male with well-documented retinitis pigmentosa. Visual acuity 20/20 OD and OS. The arterioles are normal in the posterior pole but show narrowing in the periphery. There is no evidence of pigment in the retina. Dark-adapted thresholds were elevated throughout the retina and the ERG was extinguished. *A*, fundus photograph of posterior pole area of right eye. *B*, fluorescein angiogram showing normal chorio-capillaris pattern.

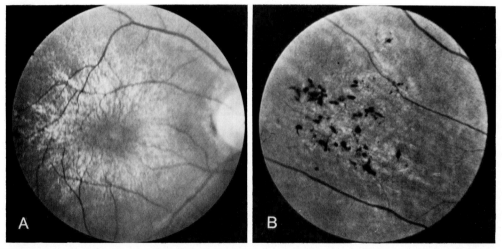

Figure 11.4 Female carrier of X-linked retinitis pigmentosa. Fundus photographs of a 48-year-old female carrier in a documented pedigree of X-linked retinitis pigmentosa. This patient had no subjective visual complaints. Visual acuity 20/20 OD and OS. Dark adaptation, EOG, and standard ERG were normal. *A*, macular area shows an unusual scintillating reflex extending around the entire parafoveal region. *B*, retinal periphery showing an isolated area of retinal pigment epithelial loss and clumps of pigment within this region.

family tree should be made, for this disorder may be inherited as autosomal recessive (AR), autosomal dominant (AD), or sex-linked recessive (X-LR). According to various studies, the percentage distribution are AR, 28–38%; AD, 12–20%; X-LR, 1–5%.[45] Most of the large group of residual unknowns in which the hereditary mode of transmission cannot be exactly defined

(simplex form) probably represent AR. A recent study in England showed somewhat different percentages more heavily weighted to the X-linked and AD varieties (AR, 15%; AD, 39%; X-LR, 25%).

In the X-linked variety of retinitis pigmentosa, the carrier female fundus shows pathognomonic changes in approximately 50% of cases (Fig. 11.4). A scintillating reflex can be seen around the foveal area, and patches of peripheral atrophy and pigment can be present. Such findings are not necessarily indicative of a widespread pathologic change. The carrier female is usually asymptomatic and will not demonstrate any obvious functional or electrical abnormalities. However, a recent study[47] has shown that the V log I function of the scotopic b-wave in carrier females has a lower slope than normal and the photopic flicker response is reduced in amplitude.

In most cases of retinitis pigmentosa, no recordable ERG response is obtained under either photopic or scotopic recording conditions. The extinguished response is *prima facie* evidence of a widespread degenerative change involving the photoreceptors. We have already noted (DG-2) that there are some forms of retinitis pigmentosa in which small amplitude responses may be recorded. This seems to occur particularly in early cases of AR retinitis pigmentosa (Fig. 11.5) as well as in the dominantly inherited (AD) mode of

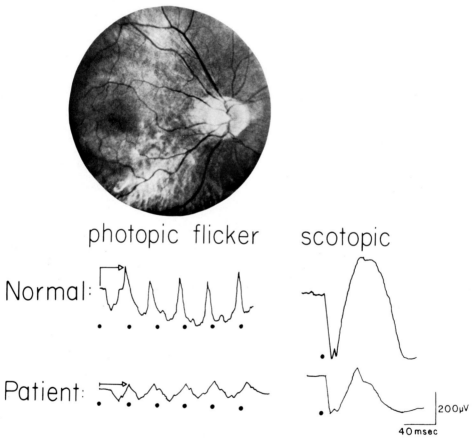

Figure 11.5 A 10-year-old boy from a family with documented autosomal recessive retinitis pigmentosa. The retina shows peripapillary myopic changes. There are scattered areas of retinal pigment epithelial loss. Occasional strands of pigment were seen in the midperiphery. The ERG shows both a decrease in amplitude and a prolonged latency (most easily seen in photopic recordings) when compared to the normal.

Dominant Retinitis Pigmentosa

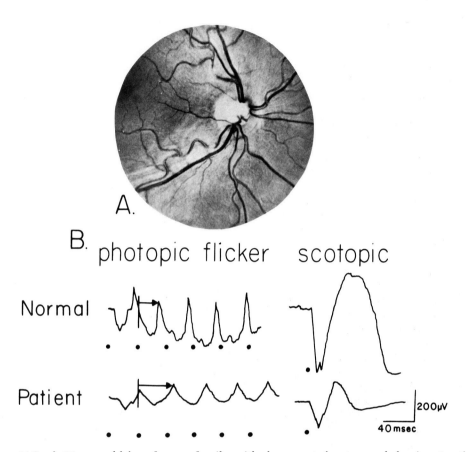

Figure 11.6 A 14-year-old boy from a family with documented autosomal dominant retinitis pigmentosa. The fundus appeared normal. Vision 20/20 OD and OS. Dark-adapted retinal thresholds are normal in the posterior pole but elevated 1.5 to 2.0 log units midperiphery. The ERGs showed a reduction in amplitude and prolonged latency. Over the course of 10 years there was a gradual accumulation of midperipheral pigment, some dropout of the pigment epithelium, and complete loss of the electrical responses under standard recording conditions.

retinitis pigmentosa in which the progress of the disorder may be much slower (Fig. 11.6). In these instances measurement of the photopic b-wave latencies may be of value.[48] Prolonged latencies in such cases will provide the additional clue for establishing the diagnosis. It should be remembered, however, that most patients with retinitis pigmentosa do not have a recordable ERG response, and latency measurements cannot be made.

ANCILLARY TEST RESULTS IN RETINITIS PIGMENTOSA

An absent response on ERG testing will go hand in hand with a very low or absent EOG light rise. We have never seen a *bona-fide* case of retinitis pigmentosa in which this was not true, but since EOG testing is much more time-consuming than the ERG, an EOG is usually not performed in cases of suspected retinitis pigmentosa.

However, the EOG may prove of value for those individuals who, because of age or corneal pathology, will not tolerate a contact lens for ERG recording. This is especially true in younger children who may be old enough to carry out the sustained eye movements required in EOG testing, yet refuse to have a contact lens electrode placed on their eye.

For all practical purposes the VEP has no place in the diagnostic evaluation of retinitis pigmentosa.

Psychophysical findings have been found to corroborate patient complaints accurately, and follow typical patterns in most instances. *Visual fields* classically show, in the early stages, a complete or partial ring scotoma which later widens to involve more peripheral and central regions; finally, in the late stages, only a small central island of vision remains. It is useful to determine field isopters with different-sized objects; in the early stages a large test object may produce an isopter of normal extent, and it is only with a small test object that a constricted field or scotomatous areas emerge.

Dark adaptometry, usually tested 15° from the fovea in the temporal or superior portions of the retina, shows elevated rod *and* cone thresholds, a further indication that this disease affects both photoreceptor types. Retinal sensitivity can also be tested at various areas throughout the retina. Thresholds thus obtained at the various retinal positions form the so-called "retinal profile," and measurements taken in areas which appear ophthalmoscopically normal may show decreased sensitivity. Such testing is more sensitive than the charting of visual fields and provides an accurate way of following patients over long periods of time.

OTHER FORMS OF GENERALIZED HEREDO-RETINAL DEGENERATIONS

There is a large group of diseases which can be considered similar to retinitis pigmentosa because they display comparable electrophysiologic and psychophysical changes. Despite their functional and symptomatic similarity to retinitis pigmentosa, these retinal degenerations display an extraordinary range of fundus alterations. When studying patients with these diseases (listed below), a detailed knowledge of the fundus appearance and mode of genetic transmission, as well as the functional findings, are essential to arrive at a correct diagnosis.

 I. Primary Retinal Abnormalities
   A. Retinitis pigmentosa sine pigmento
   B. Retinitis punctata albescens
   C. Leber's congenital amaurosis
   D. Inverse retinitis pigmentosa
   E. Progressive cone-rod degeneration
   F. Degenerative myopia
II. Primary Choroidal Abnormalities
   A. Choroideremia
   B. Gyrate atrophy of the choroid and retina
   C. Generalized choroidal sclerosis
   D. Bietti's corneo-retinal dystrophy
III. Vitreous Abnormalities and Retinoschisis
   A. X-linked recessive (vitreous veils)
   B. Autosomal dominant (Wagner)
   C. Autosomal recessive (Favré)

I. PRIMARY RETINAL ABNORMALITIES

Retinitis Pigmentosa Sine Pigmento (Fig. 11.3)

This disorder, so named because it displays none of the pigmentary changes so commonly associated with retinitis pigmentosa, can nevertheless be considered a true generalized heredo-retinal degeneration on the basis of the standard electrodiagnostic and psychophysical tests. The symptoms may be similar to those of the classic form of retinitis pigmentosa, but the absence of definitive fundus changes tends to obscure the diagnosis. The lack of retinal pigmentary abnormalities occurs during the early stages of the disease; one can expect to see more typical funduscopic changes gradually emerge with the passage of time. The necessity and importance of making the correct diagnosis as early as possible is illustrated by the following case history.

A 26-year-old white female had a 6-year history of noting blank areas in her peripheral visual field. Visual fields were difficult to obtain and were considered to be unreliable when first tested. Because of the absence of any demonstrable changes and the continuation of complaints in this very anxious woman, she was referred to a psychiatrist. One year later a visual field examination was again performed, and a temporal scotomatous region was noted. Although no x-ray abnormalities of the skull were found, an exploratory craniotomy was performed but proved to be negative. The patient then had an extreme anxiety reaction, manifested by continual complaints with regard to her vision, and she was once again referred for psychotherapy. When seen 1 year later, her fundus revealed definitely narrowed arterioles and a very fine mottled appearance. There was no evidence of any bone corpuscular pigmentary changes. Visual fields were impossible to evaluate because of poor coooperation. The suspected diagnosis of retinitis pigmentosa *sine pigmento* was borne out by the ERG, which showed an absent response.

There is little doubt that an ERG performed early in the clinical course would have immediately provided a correct diagnosis.

Retinitis Punctata Albescens (Fig. 11.7)

First described in 1882 on the basis of nightblindness and the peculiar fundus appearance, the disorder was later clarified by Lauber,[49] who in 1910 described two forms of retinitis punctata albescens: stationary and progressive. The stationary form is now known as fundus albipunctatus, a distinct type of congenital stationary nightblindness which will be discussed in detail in Chapter 14. The progressive form has characteristic fundus changes but functionally resembles retinitis pigmentosa. The retina shows slightly irregular, white, punctate lesions often dispersed throughout the fundus. The lesions are deep in the retina and can give the fundus a moth-eaten appearance. Occasionally,

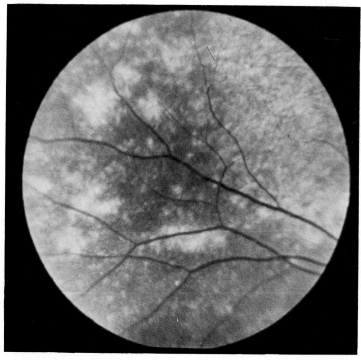

Figure 11.7 Retinitis punctata albescens. A 28-year-old male noted poor night vision and reduced side vision for 8 years. Dark-adapted thresholds were markedly elevated, and the ERG was extinguished. Both fundi showed a multitude of small, white, atrophic-appearing spots, some of which had coalesced and others of which were discrete. No overt bone-spicule pigment accumulations were seen.

pigment spicules are seen peripherally and, as is true of the generalized heredodegenerations, there is arteriolar narrowing.

In examining patients with such fundus changes it is of the utmost importance to distinguish the progressive punctata albescens form from the stationary albipunctatus form. The progressive form behaves psychophysically and electrophysiologically like a generalized retinal degeneration with elevated rod and cone thresholds, restricted visual fields, an absent or near absent ERG, and abnormal EOG light rise. As will be seen later, certain of these findings are present in fundus albipunctatus, but after a few hours in the dark, retinal functions become completely normal. The close relationship between retinitis punctata albescens and retinitis pigmentosa is further borne out by reports of the association of the two disorders in members of the same family.[50]

Leber's Congenital Amaurosis

First described by Leber[51] in 1869, the disease initially was called "amaurosis congenita." Although other names have been proposed (hereditary retinal aplasia, heredo-retinopathia congenitalis, dysgenesis neuroepithelialis retinae), the paucity and inconsistency of histologic studies argue against any change in nomenclature at present. The most recent histology study in this disorder showed primary dystrophic changes of the neurosensory retina and secondary degenerative changes in the retinal pigment epithelium and choroid.[52] The early lesions in these cases (noted as a fundus granularity) are probably produced by deposits consiting of loose outer segments, apical processes of the pigment epithelial cell, and macrophages. Other early changes are a lack of differentiation of the nuclei, the photoreceptor cells and inner segments, the pigment epithelial

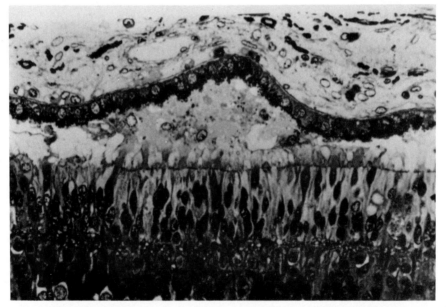

Figure 11.8 Leber's congenital amaurosis. Photomicrograph from the periphery of the right eye of a 7-month-old female whose parents were consanguineously related. Clinical findings: nystagmus was present at birth, and there was psychomotor retardation; multiple white spots with scattered pigment strands were scattered throughout the retina; ERG was extinguished; the child had frequent dyspneic episodes and died at age 18 months. The retina shows an undifferentiated pigment epithelium which is displaced from the photoreceptor layer by a subretinal deposit consisting of loose outer segments, apical processes of the pigment epithelial cells, and macrophages. The cone photoreceptors are intact, but the rods are absent. The nuclei of the outer retinal layer are undifferentiated. × 220.

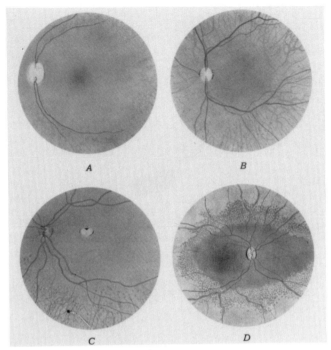

Figure 11.9 Leber's congenital amaurosis. Artist's representation of four different cases of Leber's congenital amaurosis. All patients were less than 3 years old when the fundus drawings were made. Each had psychomotor retardation with nystagmus and poor vision from birth. The ERG was extinguished in all cases. The fundus drawings show the wide range of fundus abnormalities in this particular disorder. Cases A and B showed relatively normal fundi, with the exception of the narrowed arterioles, while Cases C and D showed evident fundus changes in the macula and periphery.

cells, and the choriocapillaris (Fig. 11.8). Such widespread degenerative changes, even at the earliest stage of the disease, make it virtually impossible to delineate the exact retinal region in which the pathologic process initially occurs.

The major clinical finding in this disorder is blindness or near blindness at birth or shortly thereafter. There is often a pendular or searching nystagmus, sunken eyeballs, and photophobia. The ophthalmoscopic picture of Leber's congenital amaurosis may, however, be extremely varied[53] (Figs. 11.9 and 11.10). Several studies have reported patients whose fundi are completely normal; consistent with this finding is the result of a large study in which no ophthalmoscopically visible changes were found in 9% of the children examined.[54] Sorsby and Williams[55] found progressively severe fundus changes with advancing age associated with a wide range of retinal abnormalities in one family group.

Among the associated systemic abnormalities is a high incidence of mental retardation and generalized neuromuscular disorders. Schappert-Kimmijser and her group[54] studied 56 such children in detail. Fourteen of these patients showed major neuropsychiatric defects. It appears, therefore, that the incidence of mental retardation and often neurologic disorders in a patient with congenital amaurosis may be quite high.

When blindness in children is associated with neurologic or mental symptoms, the most common (and often erroneous) diagnosis given is blindness of "central origin." Because of the paucity of funduscopic changes in some patients with Leber's congenital amaurosis, and the difficulty of obtaining reliable subjective measures of

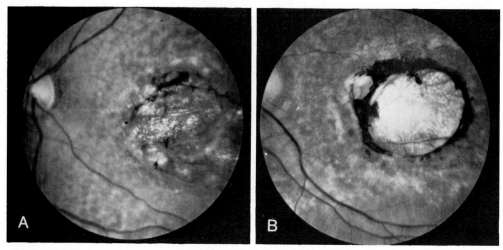

Figure 11.10 Leber's congenital amaurosis. Two siblings with deaf-mutism, poor vision, and nystagmus from birth. *A*, left eye of a 32-year-old female showing a macular coloboma, a generalized loss of the pigment epithelium and narrowed arterioles. *B*, Left eye of the 27-year-old brother with similar retinal changes. In both cases of the ERG was extinguished. Microhemagglutination testing for toxoplasmosis was negative.

retinal function, ERG results are of major diagnostic importance, and the markedly reduced or absent ERG points up the widespread abnormality of the outer retinal layers. Therefore in very young children suspected of having Leber's amaurosis, the ERG is the one method by which a firm diagnosis can be made.

This syndrome is more common than is generally realized. Schappert-Kimmijser et al.[54] in the Netherlands reported that although the incidence of this disorder in the general population is only 2 to 3 per 100,000, the incidence in a blind population was 3.8%, and in blind children it increases to 18%. An equally high incidence in blind children was also found by Alstrom and Olsen in Sweden.[56] This disorder most often occurs as an autosomal recessive, although there are reports of patients in whom the transmission may have been dominant.[57]

Inverse Retinitis Pigmentosa (Fig. 11.11)

In this disease, pigmentary changes similar to those found in the peripheral retina in typical retinitis pigmentosa appear in the macular or paramacular area only. It is important to realize that while fundus changes may indicate only a localized degenerative change, there is also the possibility that a generalized tapeto-retinal degeneration is present. The lesion may be located within the posterior pole (pericentral retinitis pigmentosa), or in the macular region itself (central retinitis pigmentosa). When the degeneration corresponds to the ophthalmoscopically affected regions, there will be corresponding scotomata, full peripheral visual fields, and an essentially normal ERG. Retinal thresholds obtained outside the affected area are normal. The mode of genetic transmission is usually given as autosomal recessive, with several instances of siblings being similarly affected.

There are also patients in whom the major ophthalmoscopic findings are confined to the central retinal area but who, in addition, show changes indicative of a generalized degeneration. This group can be considered one of the progressive cone-rod degenerations and will be described more completely in the following section. Although the ophthalmoscopic changes are located in the retinal areas far removed from those seen in typical retinitis pigmentosa, psychophysical and electrodiagnostic findings confirm the presence of a true generalized degeneration. The electroretinogram will be grossly reduced or absent, and all other tests of retinal function will be similar to retinitis pigmentosa.

Progressive Cone-Rod Degeneration

This disorder differs from typical retinitis pigmentosa in that symptoms relating to the cone system occur initially and predominate. The classification of the condition was made by Bjork et al.[58] in a group of five patients with hereditary ataxia of the Pierre-Marie type.

Patients with this disease may have no visual problems early in life; as adolescents or adults they develop signs of cone dysfunction: reduced visual acuity, lack of color sensation, and an absent or reduced photopic ERG. While visual testing reveals rod defects (elevated dark-adapted threshold and absent or markedly reduced scotopic ERGs), nonetheless in the early stages the cone abnormality exceeds that of the rods. The relative "immunity" of the macular area, usually seen early in retinitis pigmentosa, is clearly lacking in this dis-

ease. The combined rod and cone changes ultimately result not only in marked visual field constriction, but also in visual acuity far below that of the more typical forms of the generalized heredo-retinal degenerations. Because of the serious acuity deficit accompanying loss of macular function, the majority of these patients rarely mention difficulty with night vision and may actually prefer dim illumination. Both autosomal dominant or autosomal recessive modes of transmission have been reported. The following case history is illustrative of this type of disorder and points up the difficulty in arriving at the correct diagnosis.

A 32-year-old white female was referred with complaints of poor vision, photophobia, and preference for dim illumination. She felt that her poor vision was stationary since childhood, but records obtained from her physician revealed a gradual decrease in vision: 20/60 at age 8, 20/100 at age 18, and 20/200 at the time of our examination. She claimed to have no color perception at present but stated that color vision had been excellent until 20 years of age, at which time it gradually began to deteriorate.

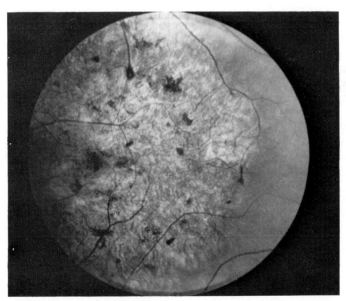

Figure 11.11 Inverse retinitis pigmentosa. A 54 year old female with poor vision for 12 years. Visual acuity 20/400 OD and OS. Both fundi are similar and show well-defined areas of pigment epithelium loss, and associated pigment strands and clumps throughout the entire macula. There is a clear demarcation from surrounding normal retina. Dark adapted thresholds were normal outside the affected-appearing retinal area. The ERG showed a reduced photopic response (with normal latencies) and a normal scotopic response.

When carefully questioned about differences in spectral hue, she was able to describe subtle color differences in support of her contention that color vision had been present at one time. Examination showed a corrected vision of OD 20/200 and OS 10/200, complete achromatopsia, markedly constricted visual fields, elevated dark thresholds from the fovea to 40° temporal and nasal retina, and an absent photopic and scotopic ERG. Ophthalmoscopy revealed a hyperpigmented macular area, moderate vascular attenuation, slight disc pallor, scattered focal areas of chorioretinal atrophy, and pigment clumps in the inferior retina of each eye (Fig. 11.12).

In this patient the functional tests indicate a widespread degenerative disorder of the photoreceptors while the history enables one to conclude that the cone system was primarily affected.

Degenerative Myopia

This disorder is included because of the degenerative retinal changes which often accompany the refractive error. Many high myopes will exhibit visual field constriction, decreased retinal sensitivity, decreased ERG amplitudes, and a reduced EOG light rise. Myopia itself, however, rarely results in extinguished electrical activity. Since myopia may also occur with generalized retinal degenerations (particularly gyrate atrophy), a reduced or absent ERG in the presence of high myopia should alert the examiner to the fact that an additional disorder is probably present.

II. PRIMARY CHOROIDAL ABNORMALITIES

Choroideremia

The only mode of inheritance known for this generalized retinal degeneration is X-linked recessive. The onset of symptoms usually occurs in the first or second decade, with the major complaint being of poor night vision.

The initial fundus appearance (Fig. 11.13A) in the affected male is a "salt-and-pepper" pigment mottling in the equator and posterior pole, and has been reported as early as age 22 months.[59] Even at this stage the ERG is abnormal, showing reduced or absent scotopic components. Below the pigment mottling, the underlying choroid may appear ophthalmoscopically normal, although fluorescein angiography may show a patchy loss of the choriocapillaris and choroidal vessels (Fig. 11.13D).

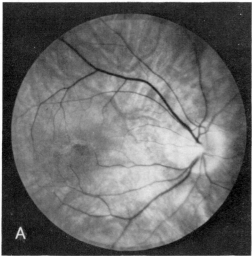 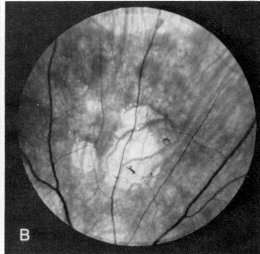

Figure 11.12   Cone-Rod degeneration. A 32-year-old white female. Description of case in text. A, macular area showing hyperpigmentation, moderate disc atrophy, and mild vascular attenuation. B, peripheral patches of depigmentation.

Later, areas of focal pigment epithelial drop out appear in the midperiphery which eventually coalesce and progress centrally; the macula is affected last, and relatively good vision is preserved until late in the disease (Fig. 11.13B). In the final stage, the entire fundus, with perhaps the exception of the macula, shows the diffuse yellowish-white reflex of the underlying sclera (Fig. 11.13C). At this stage the fundus may resemble gyrate atrophy making ophthalmoscopic distinction between the two diseases difficult. While the rate of progression may vary from individual to individual within a pedigree and also between family groups, patients with this disorder will have lost virtually all vision by age 40.

A characteristic of most x-linked diseases is that the female carrier will show specific signs; in choroideremia the fundus changes of the carrier are unique and pathognomonic of the disease. Typically, these changes superficially resemble those seen in the early stages of affected males, i.e., a generalized pigment mottling, particularly noticeable in the midperiphery and macular area (Fig. 11.13E). Despite the similar fundus appearance to the affected male, visual function is usually normal in the female and remains so throughout life. The fundus signs seen in most carriers are stationary, and fluorescein angiography shows no choriocapillaris fallout[60] (Fig. 11.13F). There are, however, some reports in which the carrier female may show some functional deficit and some abnormality on the fluorescein angiogram. The Lyon hypothesis of female mosaicism accounts for these rare occurrences.[61]

Gyrate Atrophy

Gyrate atrophy is a rare choroidal disease; it is usually inherited as an autosomal recessive disorder, although an occasional dominant pedigree has been reported. Symptoms usually appear in the 2nd and 3rd decades and consist of poor night vision and constricted visual fields. Myopia is invariably present.

The fundus abnormality begins in the midperiphery with a thinning and trans-parency of the retinal pigment epithelium; the underlying choroid may appear either normal or "sclerotic." Affected areas are separated from normal-appearing retina by scalloped borders, which begin as isolated islands which then merge to assume the form of a garland. Due to pigment accumulation, the scalloped borders have a darker appearance, thus increasing the contrast between the adjacent normal and abnormal retinal tissues (Fig. 11.14A). Fluorescein angiography shows a loss of the choriocapillaris in the affected areas (Fig. 11.14B).

As the disease progresses, pigment clumping in the retinal pigment epithelium and choriocapillaris atrophy is noted; eventually, there is disappearance of the entire choroid, exposing the white sclera. The optic disks and retinal vessels may be normal in the initial stages but later the vessels show gradual narrowing. In the very late stages choroidal atrophy may be seen from the periphery to the posterior pole, but the macula is usually spared.

Electrical and psychophysical studies indicate the presence of a generalized retinal degeneration, even in the early stages of the disorder. The late stages of gyrate atrophy may be remarkably similar to the advanced stages of choroideremia, but the different modes of genetic transmission for the two diseases is an important distinguishing factor. Also, as noted above, the female carrier in choroideremia shows distinctive funduscopic changes which help differentiate these two orders.

In 1973 Simell and Takki[62] discovered that all patients with this disorder had elevated levels of ornithine in urine and plasma. This amino acid is derived from the dietary intake of arginine. Later studies showed the elevated ornithine levels in this disorder to be due to an absence or near absence of the pyridoxine-dependent enzyme ornithine aminotransferase (OAT)[63], the catalyst necessary for the breakdown of excess ornithine in man. While it was initially felt that only the eye was affected, more recent studies have noted abnormalities in skeletal muscle and liver.[64] On the basis of these findings several patients have had a lowering of their

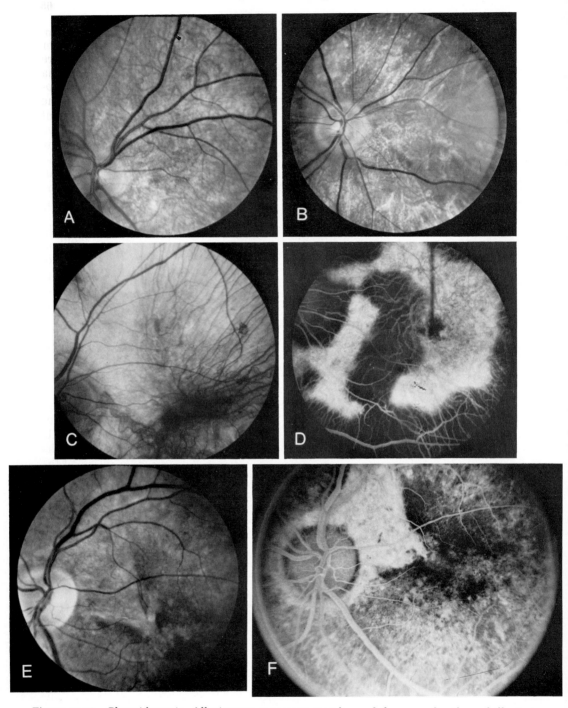

Figure 11.13 Choroideremia. All pictures represent members of the same family and illustrate the various stages of this disorder. *A*, propositus: a 10-year-old male without complaints and noted to have an unusual retinal appearance. Vision 20/20 OD and OS. The fundus shows a generalized loss of the retinal pigment epithelum and scattered small pigment clumps. His ERG was extinguished. *B*, 37-year-old maternal uncle with a history of poor night vision and reduced side vision for 20 years. Visual acuity 20/40 OD and OS. There is a marked loss of the retinal

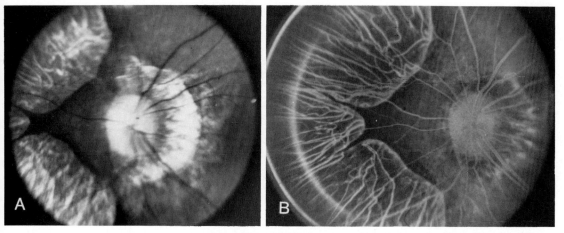

Figure 11.14 Gyrate atrophy of retina and choroid. A 39-year-old female with progressive loss of night vision and side vision. Corrected acuity: 20/70 OD and 20/80 OS. the ERG is extinguished. A, both fundi showing myopic changes around the disc. There was a scalloped border extending 360°; anterior to the border there was loss of the pigment epithelium. A hyperpigmented border separates abnormal from normal retina. B, fluorescein angiogram showing a sharp demarcation between normal and affected retina. Within the affected area there is complete loss of the choroidal pattern at the posterior border of the affected area. The patient showed a near absence of ornithine aminotransferase (OAT), but did not respond to vitamin B_6 dietary supplements.

plasma ornithine levels with vitamin B_6 alone,[65] while other patients have responded to a low-protein, low organic diet.[66] There are indications that the reduction of plasma ornithine leads to improvement in retinal function as manifested by improved dark-adapted retinal sensitivity, a slight increase in the size of the visual field, improved color discrimination, and an enhancement of the ERG response.[66]

Generalized Choroidal Dystrophy

This diffuse disorder of the choriocapillaris is usually inherited as an autosomal dominant. The onset of symptoms takes place in the 3rd and 4th decades. While symptoms of nightblindness are usually present, the symptoms associated with the photopic system (decreased vision, light aversion, photophobia) predominate.

The early fundus changes include pigment mottling, hypopigmentation, and a loss of the retinal pigment epithelium. Later, there is widespread atrophy of the retinal pigment epithelium; the choroid appears "sclerotic," with the larger vessels seen as yellowish-white streaks (Fig. 11.15A). Both the posterior pole and the periphery are involved in these changes to a varying degree, but even in the more advanced stages, the retinal vessels may be normal. In the end stages, however, this

pigment epithelium throughout the posterior pole; the periphery showed isolated patches of pigment epithelium drop out. The arterioles were generally narrowed. C, 52-year-old maternal uncle of the propositus with a severe loss of vision since age 34. There is a virtual absence of the retinal pigment epithelium and underlying choroid so that the sclera is easily visible. In the macula small areas of intact retinal pigment epithelium still persist. Visual acuity 20/400 OD and OS. D, fluorescein angiogram of 37 year old uncle showing a patchy loss of the choriocapillaris as well as intact areas of choriocapillaris. There is likewise some fallout of the large choroidal vessels. E, fundus of the 32-year-old mother; she had no ocular complaints, normal visual acuity, and no visual abnormalities on objective or subjective testing. The retina shows an unusual distribution of pigment throughout the macular area, as well as scattered clumps of pigment through the peripheral retina. F, fluorescein angiogram of the mother showing no choroidal abnormalities. The apparent blockage of fluorescein is due to pigment accumulations.

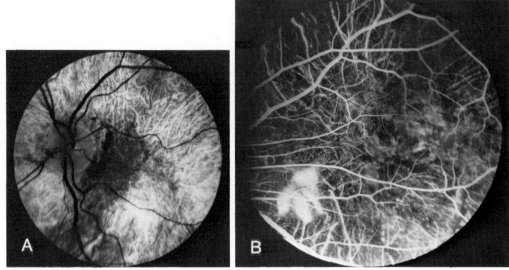

Figure 11.15 Generalized choroidal sclerosis. An 11-year-old Chinese boy whose 9 year-old-brother was similarly affected. No other family member had ocular problems. Corrected visual acuity was 5/400 OD and 20/200 OS. The ERG was extinguished. *A,* normal optic nerves and vessels. Throughout the entire retina, there was thinning and loss of the pigment epithelium associated with irregular bands and clumps of pigment. Scattered throughout the fundus were islands of normal choroid. *B,* fluorescein angiogram of the peripheral retina showing loss of the choriocapillaris associated with the areas of pigment epithelium thinning. The larger choroidal vessels were irregular in caliber and did not fill evenly.

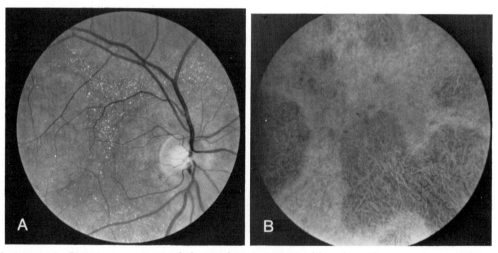

Figure 11.16 Bietti's corneo-retinal dystrophy. A 54-year-old male with no ocular complaints. Vision 20/30 OD and 20/20 OS. Visual fields showed scotomatous areas in the superior, temporal, and nasal quadrant. The photopic and scotopic ERG responses were slightly reduced; but the EOG light rise was normal. *A,* retina showing multiple, irregular, areas of pigment epithelial loss in the posterior pole. Over these regions were scattered glistening yellow-white spots. *B,* fluorescein angiography in these regions showed isolated areas of pigment epithelial loss and choriocapillaris dropout. Adjacent retinal areas appear normal.

disorder cannot be differentiated from other diffuse chorioretinal heredo-degenerations.

The psychophysical and electrophysiologic studies reflect the generalized nature of the diseaase. The ERG is either markedly subnormal or absent, while visual fields reveal varying degrees of concentric peripheral constriction.

A possible pathogenesis of this disease is indicated by fluorescein angiography, which reveals a loss of choriocapillaris and consequent visualization of the large choroidal vessels beneath the atrophic pigment epithelium (Fig. 11.15B). The severe loss of the choriocapillaris noted early in the disease leads one to consider this an abiotrophy of that particular layer.

Bietti's Corneo-Retinal Dystrophy

This rare form of heredo-degeneration shows rather specific fundus changes. The

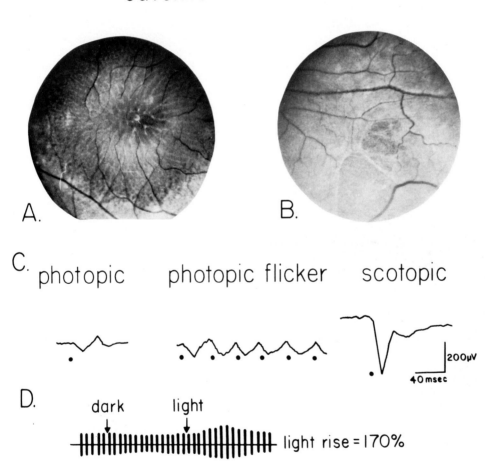

Figure 11.17 Juvenile retinoschisis. A 7-year-old male was found to have reduced vision on routine school screening. Corrected visual acuity was 20/70 OD and OS. A, macular area showing the stellate pattern macular retinoschisis. B, in the retinal periphery are seen several large lacunae with the inner retinal layers overlying them. C, ERG: the photopic response is slightly reduced in amplitude; the scotopic response is diagnostic for the disease and shows a deep negative a-wave with no b-wave. D, The EOG light rise is at the lower limits of normal; this is not considered diagnostic.

retina demonstrates varying numbers of crystalline deposits which can be noted histologically in all its layers. Scattered pigmentary changes and retinal pigment epithelial loss are also noted ophthalmoscopically (Fig. 11.16A). In addition, crystalline deposits may also be seen at the corneal limbus. A histochemical study has shown these crystals to be lipid in nature.[67] Fluorescein angiography reveals varying degrees choriocapillaris dropout (Fig. 11.16B). Related to this loss, (and its subsequent effect on photoreceptors in that particular area) the ERG and EOG will be affected to some degree. Thus, the severity of electrophysiological abnormalities mirrors the geographic loss of the choriocapillaris.

VITREOUS ABNORMALITIES AND RETINOSCHISIS

Among the more unusual forms of hereditary retinal degenerations are those in

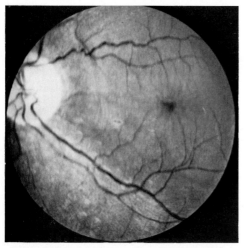

Figure 11.18   Wagner's vitreo-retinal degeneration. A 48-year-old male had poor vision for 13 years and poor night vision since his youth. One brother, his father, and his paternal grandfather had similar complaints. Both the brother and father were seen and had similar retinal changes. The fundus shows a stellate macular change and a generalized thinning of the pigment epithelium with a multitude of pigment clumps. The vitreous contained many condensed strands. Photopic and scotopic ERGs were extinguished.

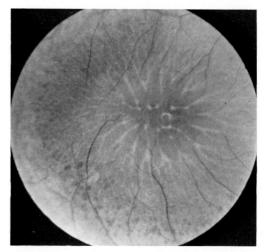

Figure 11.19   Favre's vitreo-retinal degeneration. A 17-year-old male and his 14-year-old sister had complaints of poor acuity and loss of night vision since early childhood. No other family members were so affected. The retinal changes were similar in each patient. Both demonstrated a large area of macular retinoschisis and arteriolar narrowing. Throughout the posterior pole were a multitude of small grey-black pigment clumps while the periphery of the retina showed a diffuse granularity.

which there is also a primary abnormality of the vitreous: the so-called vitreo-tapeto-retinal degenerations. Three genetic variants have been described and are clinically differentiated from each other on the basis of their ophthalmoscopic and electrophysiological findings. The test results associated with the variants overlap to such a degree that precise clinical differentiation between them is often difficult.

The sex-linked variety has a number of names but is most commonly known as either *idiopathic juvenile retinoschisis* or *congenital veils of the vitreous* (Fig. 11.17). It is found exclusively in males and characterized by macular cystic changes. In about 50% of cases an extensive peripheral retinoschisis is present, usually bilateral, in which large lacunae may be seen. The macular cysts usually do not show fluorescein leakage. The ERG is of particular importance since, in virtually all cases, the ERG shows a deep, normal a-wave and absent b-wave. The female carrier is functionally unaffected, but one study reported a possible carrier sign: large pigment clumps in isolated retinal areas.[68]

A second form, inherited as an autosomal dominant, is known as *Wagner's vitreo-retinal degeneration* (Fig. 11.18). It is characterized by an optically empty posterior vitreous, a fibrillar anterior vitreous, cataract formation, a generalized pigmentary degeneration of the retina with atrophy and sclerosis of the choroid, preretinal membranes, and as a late sequela, retinal detachment. The ERG is similar to that found in retinitis pigmentosa. Patients with this dominantly inherited variety often show facial anomalies, an association now referred to as Stickler's syndrome.[69] Some authors believe that the high frequency with which this combination of findings occurs makes the existence of two separate entities doubtful.[70]

The third and rarest of these disorders is transmitted as an autosomal recessive, and is known as *Favre's disease* (Fig. 11.19). This disorder is characterized by an optically empty vitreous with vitreo-retinal bands, pigmentary degeneration of the retina, peripheral and central retinoschisis, and at a late stage, formation of preretinal membranes. Complaints of nightblindness and an extinguished ERG are always present in this disorder.

One study[68] has emphasized that a broad range of expressivity exists within each of the three forms. Such variability may blur the distinction between forms; therefore, the mode of inheritance rather than the clinical picture, may ultimately prove to be the most important distinguishing feature.

12

Pseudo-Retinitis Pigmentosa

Certain disorders may bear an ophthalmoscopic resemblance to a generalized heredo-retinal degeneration. Because the latter diagnosis has such serious implications, every effort should be used to make certain it is correct. Often, the patient's history will help to distinguish a heredo-degenerative retinal disease from those in which the fundus picture is superficially similar. For example, a history of normal night vision and the finding of a normal dark adaptation curve are, in themselves, sufficient evidence to rule out retinitis pigmentosa. Lacking psychophysical test facilities, the electroretinogram (ERG) remains the premier test to differentiate such disorders. It has become common practice to classify those disorders listed below under the heading of pseudo-retinitis pigmentosa.

I. Infectious Diseases
   A. Viral encephalitides (i.e., rubella). Any of the childhood exanthematous disorders
   B. Disseminated chorioretinitis (i.e., syphilis)
II. Exudative Disorders
   A. Harada's disease (after resolution of exudative detachments)
   B. Toxemia of pregnancy (after resolution of detachment)
III. Drug-induced Retinal Degenerations
   A. Phenothiazines
   B. 4-Amino quinolines
IV. Exogenous Causes
   A. Ophthalmic artery occlusion
   B. Trauma
   C. Metallosis
V. Miscellaneous
   A. Uniocular retinitis pigmentosa
   B. Sectoral retinitis pigmentosa
   C. Pericentral retinitis pigmentosa
   D. Paravenous retinal distrophy
   E. Fundus flavimaculatus

INFECTIOUS DISEASES

The disseminated retinitis found in rubella as well as in other viral encephalitides shows a characteristic salt-and-pepper distribution of pigment throughout the retina (Fig. 12.1). Retinal function, however, is not compromised, and the ERG is normal. Since systemic abnormalities such as deafness or mental retardation may also occur in rubella, as well as in some forms of retinitis pigmentosa, this syndrome-complex may be confusing to the examiner. Thus, in children from whom psychophysical data cannot be obtained, the electrodiagnostic tests of retinal function remain the prime diagnostic modality.

Certain disseminated chorioretinitides may give abnormal ERG responses which are indicative of the amount of retina affected. At one extreme, infectious diseases involving most of the retina can lead to an extinguished ERG. In such cases, the diagnostic differentiation from retinitis pigmentosa may be difficult, if not impossible. Helpful diagnostic points in such cases are the history of prior good night vision, the onset of a suspected inflammatory process, asymmetry between the two eyes, and most importantly, determination of the b-wave latency (if any ERG is present). A normal time to peak of the b-wave is commonly found in chorioretinitis, but is increased in most cases of retinitis pigmentosa.

EXUDATIVE DISORDERS

Harada's disease, as well as toxemia of pregnancy, may lead to an exudative detachment, which after resolving may result in a heavily pigmented area outlining the

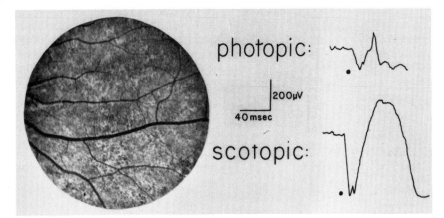

Figure 12.1 Chorioretinitis (rubella). A 12-year-old male with deafness and no ocular complaints. The mother had rubella during pregnancy. The retina showed a scattering of pigment throughout with associated patchy loss of the retinal pigment epithelium. The ERG was normal, indicating no generalized abnormality of the photoreceptors.

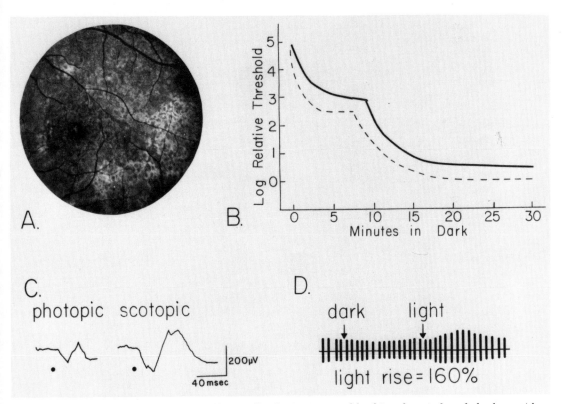

Figure 12.2 Drug-induced retinopathy (Mellaril). A 23-year-old schizophrenic female had a rapid loss of vision occurring over a period of 3 months. She had been hospitalized the prior year and was on multiple medications. She had been on Mellaril (1200 mg/day), for a period of 8 months. Her corrected visual acuity was 20/100 OD and 20/200 OS. A, fundi similar to each other and showed large clumps of pigment throughout the retina but most marked in the posterior pole. B, Course of dark adaptation compared to a normal (*dashed line*), showing a mild elevation of both cone and rod thresholds. C, ERG reduced for all conditions of stimulation. D, EOG light rise also reduced (normal = >180%).

previous detachment. Often, the history will suffice to differentiate such disorders from the generalized heredo-retinal degenerations. The ERG can be helpful; it will be reduced in amplitude but latency measurements will be normal, reflecting the fact that those regions of the retina contributing to the response are normal.

DRUG-INDUCED RETINAL DEGENERATION

Certain types of drugs are known to produce generalized retinal degenerations; both the 4-amino quinolines, as well as the phenothiazines, are typical examples. They both are taken up readily by mela-

nin-containing cells, with the highest uptake occurring in the pigment epithelium of the retina. The tight binding of these substances within these pigmented cells, along with the very slow excretion rate, produces a buildup of these materials in the retina, which in turn interferes with the metabolic processes of the pigment epithelium and leads ultimately to degenerative changes of the photoreceptor-pigment epithelial complex.[71]

The *phenothiazines* are well-known agents which produce toxic retinopathy. Indeed, it was the resultant retinopathy which prompted the removal of the experimental drug NP-207 from the market.[72] Since then, other drugs of this genre, notably, Mellaril (Thioridazine), have been

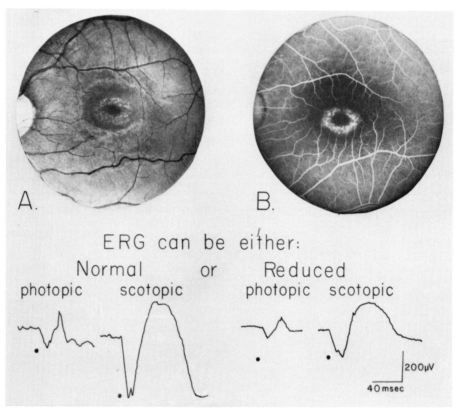

Figure 12.3 Chloroquine retinopathy. A 14-year-old boy was taking chloroquine for leprosy. He took a daily dose of 500 mg for a total dose of approximately 940 g. His visual acuity was 20/20 in each eye. A, fundus showing typical bullseye within the macular area. B, fluorescein angiogram showing a well-circumscribed circle of pigment epithelial loss with surrounding hyperpigmentation. The foveal area is normal. The ERG in this particular case was normal, although cases similar to this may have a reduced response. Some patients may go on to a generalized retinal degeneration with an associated extinguished ERG.

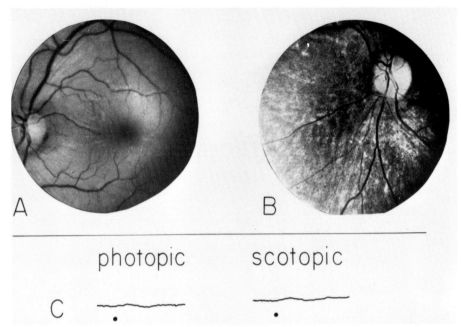

Figure 12.4 Ophthalmic artery occlusion. A 23-year-old female had gas anesthesia delivered through a face mask during cesarean section. One hour after delivery she noted loss of light perception in her left eye. *A*, fundus evaluation showing generalized edema of the retina and a cherry red spot. *B*, six months later generalized loss of the pigment epithelium, a scattering of large clumps of pigment throughout the retina, narrowed arterioles, and a pale disc. *C*, ERG in the acute phase extinguished, indicating loss of the vascular supply to both the outer and the inner retinal layers.

implicated. The retinal degenerative changes seem dose related; a high ingestion rate over several months is necessary to produce the defects. The retinal changes may occur slowly over a period of several months, and in severe cases a dense mottling of pigment may appear throughout the retina (Fig. 12.2).

Chloroquine and its congeners have been known to produce a variety of retinal disturbances.[73] While the localized macular bullseye lesion is the most commonly seen retinal abnormality (Fig. 12.3), some individuals may progress to a generalized type of pigmentary degeneration. Indeed, even after cessation of medication there may be further retinal damage, again because of the very slow excretion rate of these drugs.[74]

While both the phenothiazines and the chloroquine derivatives show fundus features not particularly typical of the heredoretinal degenerations, certain cases will show electrodiagnostic changes consistent with a generalized degeneration. On the other hand, contrary to some early studies,[75] neither the electrooculogram (EOG) nor the ERG is a reliable index of *early* retinal dysfunction produced by chloroquine. While there may be some statistically significant decrements in b-wave amplitudes when comparing a large number of chloroquine patients with a normal population, such results have little value as reliable predictors of early retinal changes when evaluating the individual patient. Of course, a gross ERG abnormality is indeed an unequivocal indication of severe retinal change, and if electrical responses are markedly reduced the medication should be immediately stopped.

EXOGENOUS CAUSES

Among the miscellaneous group of diseases which may show a fundus picture

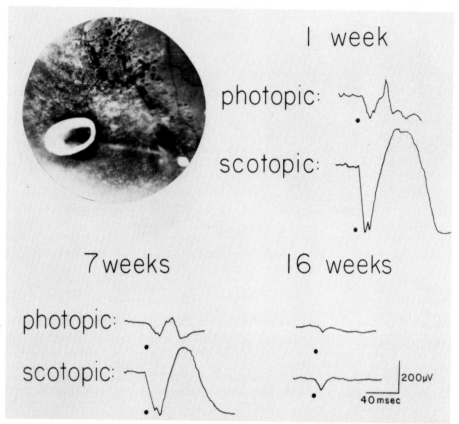

Figure 12.5 Metallosis (siderosis bulbi): Iron. A 16-year-old boy was chipping at a block of wood with an ax when the ax hit an underlying piece of metal and a sharp object hit the eye. There was slight local pain around the eye, but this was transient. One week later the boy was brought to the hospital. A metallic foreign body was localized in front of the retina in the infero-temporal quadrant. An ERG at this time was normal. Surgery was refused. Seven weeks after the accident, the boy was seen again, and the ERG showed a generalized reduction in amplitude. Again, surgery was refused. At 16 weeks, marked pigmentary changes were noted around the site of the foreign body, and a generalized granularity was seen throughout the retina. The ERG now showed only a small negative response. At this time, the foreign body was uneventfully removed, but the patient was lost to follow-up.

similar to retinitis pigmentosa, two are easily distinguished since they are unilateral: ophthalmic artery occlusion and trauma.

Occlusion of the ophthalmic artery, usually reported as occurring after compression from face mask anesthesia,[76] initially produces a picture similar to central retinal artery occlusion, but later there is generalized retinal atrophy, pigment clumping, and optic atrophy (Fig. 12.4). Since there is virtually total destruction of the outer retinal layers through loss of the choroidal blood supply, the ERG is absent from the earliest stage.

Traumatic injuries to an eye can also lead to changes similar to those just described for vascular insult. The history as well as the presence of a normal fellow eye will, of course, distinguish both of these problems from retinitis pigmentosa.

ERG occupies a unique position in the study of *intraocular foreign bodies* (Fig. 12.5). While radiography and ultrasonography are no doubt of greater importance in localization of a foreign body, ERG testing may be used to determine if an intraocular foreign body is causing retinal damage and should be removed.

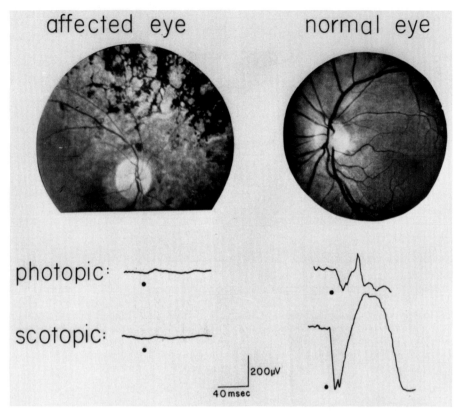

affected eye   normal eye

photopic:

scotopic:

200μV

40 msec

Figure 12.6 Uniocular retinitis pigmentosa. A 47-year-old male had been followed for 16 years with an unchanging retinal picture. When initially seen by the referring ophthalmologist at age 26, he had complaints of flashes of light in the right eye. Vision was 20/20 OD and OS. The left fundus was normal in appearance. The right eye showed disc pallor, narrowed arterioles, and heavy pigment accumulation throughout the peripheral retina. The ERG was extinguished in the right eye and normal in the left eye. Follow-up studies have shown a gradual reduction in acuity of the affected eye to 20/200 and increasing granularity in the macular area; the peripheral retina appeared unchanged. The left eye has remained normal in all respects.

Not all foreign bodies may lead to retinal cellular damage and such factors as the nature of the metal, its alloy content, intraocular localization, and duration are factors which influence the development of metallosis. The most common foreign bodies causing retinal degeneration are those containing iron and copper, although aluminum may also be damaging. These ions are also toxic when present in alloys; the percentage present is an obvious factor of importance.

The ERG findings are rather typical, although there are a number of references in the literature to an initial period in which the entire ERG is abnormally large (i.e.,

supernormal ERG). In our experience, the ERG findings are rather typical and are similar to those reported by Knave.[77] The initial change is an abnormally large a-wave and reduced b-wave. Subsequently, there is further loss of the b-wave. The a-wave then becomes reduced until electrical silence signals massive retinal cellular degeneration. Restitution of normal responses may occur if the foreign body is removed before the a-wave is affected. This would indicate in man that the initial dissemination of ions is through the inner retinal layers, with later changes involving the photoreceptors.[78]

One question which arises is how long

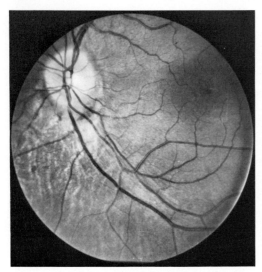

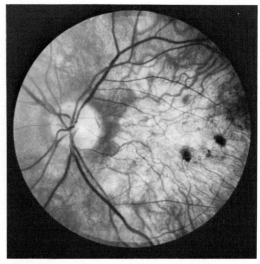

Figure 12.7 Sectorial retinitis pigmentosa. A 40-year-old male with no ocular complaints. There was a wedge-shaped pattern of pigment epithelial loss involving the inferonasal quadrant of the retina in both eyes. Several groups of pigment spicules were located within the affected area. The ERG was normal.

Figure 12.9 Central retinitis pigmentosa. A 37-year-old white male with vision 20/30 OD and hand movements OS. Both fundi show a loss of pigment, with pigment clumping within the affected macular area. A small area around the fovea of the right eye is spared. An ERG showed reduced photopic responses and normal scotopic responses.

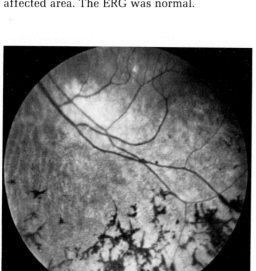

Figure 12.8 Retinitis pigmentosa with sectorial pigment changes. An 18-year-old black female with a complaint of poor night vision for 6 years. Both retinas showed mild granularity of the entire fundus, but the major ophthalmoscopic change was a large wedge-shaped area in the inferior retina with heavy bone-spicule pigmentation. Despite the localized fundus abnormality, the ERG was absent.

to follow a patient with a retained intraocular foreign body if the ERG is normal. A review of the literature shows that 3–4 months is a sufficient period of time. If changes are not evident by that time, it is unlikely that they will appear in the future.

MISCELLANEOUS

All the types of so-called atypical retinitis pigmentosa are distinguishable on the basis of history, fundus appearance, and the ERG responses. *Uniocular retinitis pigmentosa* (Fig. 12.6), presents a classic picture of retinitis pigmentosa in one eye only. It has never been reported to have a familial occurrence, and there are perfectly normal findings in the fellow eye. This asymmetric disorder may have as its etiology a slow occlusive process involving the ophthalmic and/or short posterior ciliary arteries[76] or a slowly evolving neuroretinitis.[79]

Sectorial retinitis pigmentosa is an unusual disorder, in which the fundus shows

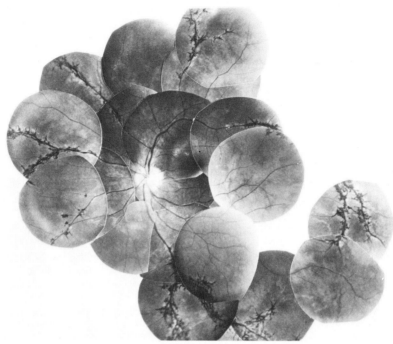

Figure 12.10 Paravenous chorioretinal dystrophy. A 23-year-old male with normal acuity and no ocular complaints. On routine fundus evaluation, paravenous deposits of pigment were noted, particularly in the midperipheral area. The ERG was normal.

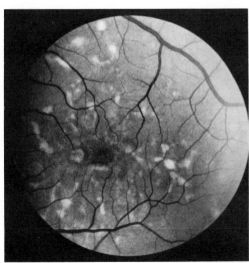

Figure 12.11 Fundus flavimaculatus. A 16-year-old white male with corrected acuity of 20/60 OD and OS. A 12-year-old sister was reported to have macular degeneration. The macular area has a granular appearance. Scattered throughout the entire posterior pole were multiple irregular yellow-white lesions, most with indistinct borders.

a wedge-shaped area, usually located inferonasally in each eye, which appears ophthalmoscopically similar to retinitis pigmentosa (Fig. 12.7). Though few pedigrees exist, it is considered to be genetically transmitted as an autosomal dominant. All test results obtained in the uninvolved retinal areas are normal—an important diagnostic finding. Since only a small region of the retina is actually affected, the standard ERG and the EOG will be normal. Likewise, dark adaptation, performed *outside* of the visibly disturbed region, will be normal. It is of utmost importance to perform retinal electrical testing in such patients since there exist varieties of a generalized retinal degeneration in which the sole pigmentary changes at an early stage are present only in circumscribed areas (Fig. 12.8). However, in the latter instances, a grossly abnormal ERG will point to the correct diagnosis.

Pericentral retinitis pigmentosa is a term used for a macular degenerative change in which there are pigmentary deposits within the macula resembling the strands of bone-corpuscular pigment seen in true retinitis pigmentosa (Fig. 12.9). Since this is a localized degeneration the ERG and EOG will be normal as will retinal sensitivity measures obtained in the periphery of the dark adapted retina.

Paravenous retinal dystrophy is a rare disorder of unknown cause but the retinal picture is quite diagnostic (Fig. 12.10). Alongside some of the retinal veins runs a track of pigment. The pigment clumps will often have a bone-corpuscular configuration. The ERG is normal or only slightly affected in this disease, the sole abnormality being enlarged angioscotomata reflecting the limited retinal disturbance in the vicinity of the vessels. There has recently been some evidence that this disorder may be slowly progressive.[80] The

disorder of *fundus flavimaculatus* can be a source of diagnostic difficulty. It is a hereditary macular degeneration which often shows scattered yellow-white spots outside of the macula and occasionally throughout the retina (Fig. 12.11). Pigment strands in the peripheral retina are also noted in some cases. Pathologic evaluation has shown that the atrophic-appearing yellow spots are accumulations of a PAS-positive material lying at the basal portion of the pigment epithelial cells, and they themselves are not indicative of any retinal dysfunction.[81] A more recent study has demonstrated a heavy accumulation of lipofuscin within the pigment epithelium.[82] The ERG and tests of peripheral retinal sensitivity are normal, a further indication that the greater portion of the retina is normal.

13

Generalized Heredoretinal Degenerations Associated with Systemic Diseases

Studying the association of various sorts of retinal degeneration with specific systemic disorders, many of which are listed in Table 13.1, is a speciality in itself. Such studies are not, however, academic, since uncovering an association may often point to causative factors underlying the various forms of hereditary retinal degenerations.

BASSEN-KORNZWEIG SYNDROME

Patients with Bassen-Kornzweig syndrome, first described in 1950,[83] may show malformed erythrocytes (acanthocytosis), neuromuscular disturbances with ataxia, fat intolerance, and retinitis pigmentosa. The funduscopic changes described in some of the reported cases range from the typical fundus picture of retinitis pigmentosa to one which more closely resembles that of retinitis punctata albescens. Strabismus and associated nystagmus have also been seen in several patients and may well be related to the central nervous system defect. All psychophysical and electroretinographic findings are quite similar to those seen in the generalized retinal degenerations.

Although this disorder was initially believed to be due to an absence of β-lipoprotein,[84] later evidence revealed that other lipoproteins were also reduced.[85] In addition to low serum fat and cholesterol, there is a concomitant lowering of the fat-soluble vitamins, including vitamin A. Recent studies have shown that vitamin A supplements in sufficient dose to normal-ize the serum vitamin A also produce normal dark-adapted thresholds and an increase of the previously reduced ERG.[86] It is not known, however, if the vitamin A acts directly on the dystrophic retinal tissue or whether it restores the low rhodopsin content of the receptor, thus secondarily increasing receptor function. In any case, the reversal of retinal degeneration with administration of large doses of vitamin A indicates that the Bassen-Kornzweig syndrome may be a treatable form of retinal degeneration.

In several respects, the clinical course of the retinal changes in this condition resembles that of severe vitamin A deficiency. For example, in both conditions, rod vision deteriorates at an earlier stage than cone vision. This is thought to be due to the fact that cone visual pigments are synthesized less rapidly than rod pigments, so that when vitamin A is in short supply the needs of the cones are satisfied more effectively than those of the rods.

In order to establish whether vitamin A deficiency alone is responsible for the retinal degeneration in the Bassen-Kornzweig syndrome, it is important to maintain normal serum vitamin A levels in such patients from the earliest possible age, and to monitor retinal sensitivity with psychophysical tests as well as the ERG.

REFSUM'S SYNDROME

Refsum's syndrome (heredopathia atactica polyneuritiformis), first described in

81

Table 13.1
Specific Systemic Disorders

Disorder	Signs and symptoms
Metabolic Disorders	
A. Lipid abnormalities	
1. Bassen-Kornzweig (AR)	Acanthocytosis; cerebellar ataxia; celiac disease
2. Refsum (AR)	Polyneuropathy; ataxia; increased CSF protein
3. Hooft (AR)	Skin rash; mental retardation; growth retardation
B. Ceroid lipofuscinosis	
1. Battens (AR)	Mental retardation, seizures; loss of motor coordination
2. Hallervorden-Spatz (AR)	Basal ganglia symptoms, dementia
C. Mucopolysaccharoidoses	
1. MPS-I-H: Hurler (AR)	Skeletal abnormalities; cloudy corneas; mental retardation
2. MPS-I-S: Scheie (AR)	Broad facies; cloudy corneas, normal intelligence
3. MPS-II: Hunter (XLR)	Skeletal abnormalities; hepatosplenomegaly; mental retardation
4. MPS-III: Sanfilippo (AR)	Mental retardation
Neurologic Diseases	
A. Friedreich's ataxia (AR)	Posterior column disease; nystagmus; ataxia
B. Marie's ataxia (AD)	Cerebellar ataxia
C. Usher (AR)	Deafness
D. With ophthalmoplegia (?)	Ataxia; cardiac abnormalities; ocular myopathy
E. Laurence-Moon (AR)	Mental retardation; hypogenitalism
F. Bardet-Biedl (AR)	Mental retardation; hypogenitalism; obesity; polydactyly
G. Rare associations	
1. Flynn-Aird (AD)	Cataracts; ataxia; dementia; epilepsy; skin lesions
2. Pelizaeus-Merzbacher (XLR)	Spasticity, cerebellar ataxia; mental retardation
3. With pallidal degeneration (AR)	Extrapyramidal rigidity; dysarthria
Miscellaneous Rare Associations	
A. Familial Nephropathies (AR) Alport; Fanconi	Renal failure
B. Alagille (AR)	Liver disease; obesity; mental retardation
C. Marfan (AD)	Skeletal abnormalities; subluxated lenses; cardiac disorders
D. Alstrom (AR)	Obesity, diabetes mellitus
E. Cockayne (AR)	Dwarfism; nanism; mental retardation
F. With megacolon (Polygenic)	Polar cataracts; strabismus
G. Turner (Chromosomal)	Infertility, short stature; webbed neck
H. Kartagener (AR)	Dextrocardia; bronchiectasis
I. With retinal vascular disease	Retinal angiomata (Coats) Peripheral neovascularization

1946,[87] is an autosomal recessive disorder predominantly affecting the nervous system. The characteristic eye findings in this syndrome are an atypical retinitis pigmentosa with nightblindness and constriction of the visual fields; neurological signs include chronic polyneuritis with progressive paresis of the distal parts of the extremities, elevated cerebrospinal fluid protein, and ataxia with other cerebellar signs. Less frequently seen are anosmia, pupillary abnormalities, cataracts, deafness, alterations of the ECG, and skeletal abnormalities.

Nightblindness is present in nearly all patients studied and is the most common initial ocular symptom. Associated with the nightblindness are constriction of the visual fields and abnormal fundus pigmentation. The retinal pigmentation is usually a mottled, nondescript type, although typical bone corpuscular configuration has sometimes been observed. Such findings are sufficient to make the clinical diagnosis of retinitis pigmentosa. The results of electroretinographic studies of patients with Refsum's disease are consistent with a generalized retinal degeneration.

In 1963, abnormal levels of a long-chain fatty acid were detected in the serum, urine, kidney, and liver of a patient with Refsum's disease.[88] This fatty acid, 3,7,11,15-tetramethylhexadecanoic (phytamic acid) was subsequently found in other patients with this syndrome. An interesting relationship has been suggested between the presence of this fatty acid and the associated atypical retinitis pigmentosa. Baum et al.[89] hypothesized that since palmitic acid, found in its esterified form at high concentrations in normal retina, is structurally similar to phytamic acid, there may be a competitive interference between the two which may disturb fatty acid metabolism concerned with the esterification of palmitic acid and retinol in the dark phase of the rhodopsin cycle.

Patients whose serum phytamic acid levels were lowered by means of a low phytamic acid diet showed remarkable improvement in their neurologic status.[90] There was no mention of the ocular findings in these patients, but such therapy should be entertained in an attempt to either halt or improve the retinal degenerative changes.

HOOFT'S DISEASE

This disorder, originally described in 1962,[91] is a syndrome-complex which demonstrates a slight growth retardation, an erythematous squamous skin eruption, mental retardation, a generalized retinal degeneration, hypolipidemia, hypocholesterolemia, and hypophospholipidemia. The specific enzymic defect producing the metabolic abnormalities is not yet known, but it is considered to be one of the forms of metachromatic leukodystrophies.

NEURONAL CEROID LIPOFUSCINOSES

These diseases were originally included under the classification of the "amaurotic familial idiocies," a term introduced by Sachs to designate a group of disorders with cerebral and retinal abnormalities and mental retardation. Later investigations led to a subdivision of amaurotic familial idiocy into six different forms with an array of eponyms which has led to a great deal of confusion regarding the interrelationship of the various types. Two of the forms within the subgroup of amaurotic familial idiocy are associated with a generalized heredo-retinal degeneration. The most common of these is now known as Batten's disease or neuronal ceroid lipofucinosis to delinate the biochemical changes. In the past the disease was known as Vogt-Spielmeyer or Batten-Mayou Disease. An adult form of ceroid lipofuscinosis is also recognized and was formerly known as Kufs' disease (adult amaurotic idiocy) or, more recently, Hallervorden-Spatz disease. Further study has uncovered more subcategories, but for our purposes it is sufficient to be aware that all of the neuronal ceroid lipofuscinoses are progressive diseases which lead to mental and motor degeneration, as well as severe visual loss. The onset is usually slow and can occur during infancy or childhood with the rate of progression and time of onset varying in the different types. In all the different varieties, the ophthalmoscopic findings are similar and include atrophic discs, a brownish hyperpigmentation in the macular area, and generalized degenerative changes throughout the retina which histologically appear to be a combination of abnormalities of the ganglion cell and photoreceptor layers.[92]

MUCOPOLYSACCHARIDE (MPS) ABNORMALITIES

These disorders include the following, biochemically separable, varieties: MPS-I-

H (Hurler's disease, gargolyism, dysostosis multiplex); MPS I-S (Scheie's syndrome); MPS II (Hunter's syndrome); MPS III, (Sanfilippo's syndrome); MPS IV, (Morquio's syndrome); and MPS VI (Maroteaux-Lamy syndrome). These disorders may be distinguished by the presence (I-S, IV) or absence (I-H, II, VI) of corneal clouding, the degree of behavioral aberrations (worst in III), and the type of mucopolysaccharide excreted in the urine. Four of the varieties, PMS I-H, I-S, II, and III show abnormal ERGs. This finding and the results of other testing indicate the presence of generalized tapetoretinal degenerations in the majority of such patients. Sidman[93] found MPSs in the interstitial matrix of the outer segments of the rods and cones; thus, abnormalities of MPS metabolism may have a primary deleterious effect on visual receptor cell metabolism.

NEUROLOGIC DISORDERS

While a number of neurologic disorders are frequently associated with a tapetoretinal degeneration, two of the earliest recognized were the *Laurence-Moon* and *Bardet-Biedl* syndromes. This separation into two distinct disorders is more in keeping with what was initially described by each of the original groups. Laurence and Moon noted retinal degeneration with hypogenitalism and mental retardation, while the complete syndrome, i.e., including the additional associations of deafness and polydactyly, was described by Bardet and Biedl. Of the multiple abnormalities associated with this disorder, generalized retinal degeneration is the most common, being found in 90–95% of the cases. In many of these patients, macular degeneration is an early occurrence. Ophthalmoscopic changes in the peripheral retina may be minimal, so the electrodiagnostic findings of reduced ERG a- and b-waves will often be the only clue to the existence of a widespread loss of retinal function.

Among the hereditary ataxias, two main types are distinguished. *Friedreich's ataxia*, which appears between ages 6 and 25, produces cerebellar abnormalities in gait and hand movements, profound sensory disturbances, and later, trophic disturbances. *Marie's ataxia* usually begins at about age 25; it also results in severe cerebellar signs, but there is an exaggeration of the tendon reflexes with clonus.

In both forms of ataxia, a generalized tapetoretinal degeneration may occur. This is observed more frequently in Marie's than in Friedreich's ataxia, but both forms have well-documented cases of the association. Each form may also show macular degenerative changes accompanying the generalized degeneration. The wide range of expressivity manifested by some patients with Friedreich's ataxia is well-illustrated in the study of Franceschetti and Klein.[94] In this pedigree, among the 21 members with ataxia, there were six with macular degeneration, four with pigmentary retinopathy, and two with retinitis punctata albescens, hence, the necessity for complete visual testing if the proper diagnosis and prognosis are to be accurately assigned.

Progressive external ophthalmoplegia may be associated with a diffuse pigmentary disturbance of the retina. Rarely, however, has this retinopathy been reported to produce an abnormal ERG. The ophthalmoplegia will usually bring such patients to the attention of the examiner. While the ocular myopathy is progressive, the fundus changes do not seem to worsen along with the neurological deficit. Kearns and coworkers[95] added the observation that in addition to retinal changes with external ophthalmoplegia, there is also cardiomyopathy, the latter complication leading to death from heart block in some cases. Therefore, a patient with external ophthalmoplegia and retinal changes should also be referred for cardiac evaluation.

14

Congenital Stationary Nightblindness

The group of disorders known collectively as congenital stationary nightblindness (CSNB) can, because of patient symptoms, be confused with a generalized heredo-retinal degeneration. Making the distinction even more difficult is the fact that the electroretinogram (ERG) is abnormal in all forms of CSNB. However, the configuration of the ERG response itself will, in addition to results of other procedures, help the examiner to make the correct diagnosis. These night-blinding diseases can be conveniently partitioned as follows:

I. CSNB with normal fundi (AD, AR, X-LR)
II. CSNB with abnormal fundi
    Oguchi's disease (AR)
    Fundus albipunctatus (AR)
III. CSNB with myopia, nystagmus, and decreased vision (X-LR)

CSNB WITH NORMAL FUNDI

This most common form of CSNB may be inherited as an autosomal recessive (AR), autosomal dominant (AD), or X-linked recessive (X-LR). The fundus picture is completely normal, as are visual fields, two key findings allowing differentiation between CSNB and retinitis pigmentosa. Compared to the usual two-branched (cone and rod) dark adaptation curve seen in normals, these CSNB patients have only the cone branch which attains essentially normal threshold levels, a circumstance rarely seen in retinitis pigmentosa.

The ERG findings permit separation of two forms of CSNB with normal fundi; both have similar dark adaptometry functions and can only be distinguished by comparing the results of electrical testing.

The most common form (type 1) has a negative ERG (no b-wave) in scotopic or photopic levels of adaptation but a normal electrooculogram (EOG) (Fig. 14.1). The other (type 2) has a markedly attenuated ERG; both a- and b-waves are reduced under all test conditions (Fig. 14.2). In addition, this latter form of CSNB has an abnormally low EOG light rise. Were it not for the normal fundus, the normal latency of the cone ERG responses, and normal cone threshold, the type 2 variety of CSNB could easily be confused with a generalized retinal degeneration.

It is possible, knowing the origins of the a- and b-wave components of the ERG and the light rise of the EOG, to formulate a hypothesis regarding the lesion site of these two forms of CSNB. Since fundus reflectometric data unequivocally show that rhodopsin concentration and its regeneration kinetics are normal for both of these forms of CSNB, abnormalities in the electrical properties of neural transmission must somehow account for the observed findings.[96]

For the type 1 CSNB, the lack of a b-wave with normal a-wave and normal EOG light rise would place the lesion in the region of the bipolar cells, but close to the outer plexiform layer. The second type, lacking normal a- and b-wave voltages, *as well as* having a reduced EOG light rise, implicates neural activity deriving from more distal regions, possibly involving the inner segments of the receptors themselves (see Chapters 2 and 9).

CSNB WITH ABNORMAL FUNDI

In *Oguchi's disease* (Fig. 14.3), the retina has a peculiar silvery metallic sheen with

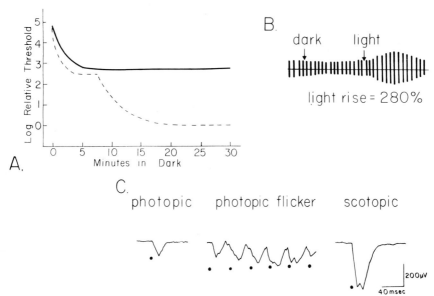

Figure 14.1 CSNB with normal fundus (type I). A 19-year-old male with complaints of poor night vision all of his life. Visual acuity was 20/20 OD and OS. *A*, dark adaptation curve comparing the patient (*solid line*) with the normal (*dashed line*). The affected patient shows no evidence of rod adaptation, but the cone recovery portion of the function is near normal. *B*, normal EOG light rise. *C*, ERG showing only a negative (a-wave) response of normal amplitude, with no positive component.

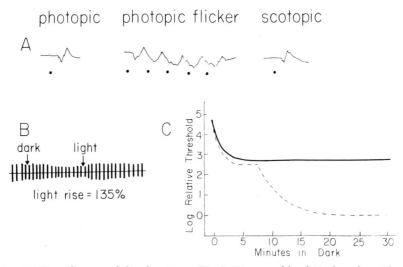

Figure 14.2 CSNB with normal fundus (type II). A 32-year-old white female with poor night vision all of her life. There is a family history of night blindness; her father and one sister, as well as one of her sister's sons, were similarly affected. *A*, ERG showing a small brisk response under photopic conditions which remains unchanged in the dark. *B*, EOG showing an abnormal light rise. *C*, patient's dark adaptation (*solid line*) shows no evidence of rod adaptation compared to the normal (*dashed line*). There is a very slight elevation in the cone portion of the curve.

the retinal vessels standing out in marked contrast and appearing quite dark. This unusual picture can be seen throughout the retina or may just be found in the posterior pole or periphery. These retinal changes should provide a sufficient clue to the diagnosis, but several other related findings are also important. If the patient is kept in total darkness for a few hours, the peculiar retinal sheen will disappear (Mizuo's phenomenon); at the end of this time the patient will also have achieved normal dark-adapted thresholds.[97] There is no known association between the slow dark adaptation rate and the change in fundus coloration, but these unusual findings are differential points which can be critical in making the correct diagnosis.

The ERG is abnormal after 30 minutes of dark adaptation; it shows a normal a-wave but an absent b-wave. After prolonged dark adaptation (approximately 3 hours) at a time when thresholds have reached normal levels, the ERG, in most cases, continues to show only a normal a-wave. In some cases, under certain recording conditions a fully developed b-wave can be elicited.[98] This disorder also shows normal visual pigment concentration and kinetics. The pathogenesis seems due to some as yet unknown abnormality in neural transmission in the retina.[99]

The second disorder in this group, fundus albipunctatus (Fig. 14.4), is often confused with the progressive generalized degeneration known as retinitis punctata al-

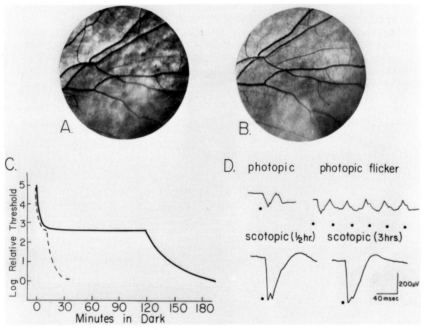

Figure 14.3 Oguchi's disease. A 29-year-old male has had problems with dark adaptation all of his life. He did note, however, that after prolonged periods in the dark, his sensitivity appeared normal. A brother is similarly affected. *A*, appearance of the retina following light adaptation. There is a metallic sheen to the entirety of the retina, with the retinal vessels standing out in dark relief against this unusual background. *B*, same area of the retina following 3 hours of dark adaptation, appearing normal with disappearance of the unusual metallic reflex. *C*, recovery of dark adaptation followed over a period of 180 minutes. The patient (*solid line*) is compared to the normal (*dashed lines*). The cone system quickly attains normal sensitivity levels, but the rods reach normal thresholds only after 3 hours. *D*, ERG showing essentially only an a-wave with a reduced b-wave under scotopic and photopic conditions. There is little change in the ERG waveform, even after 3 hours of adaptation.

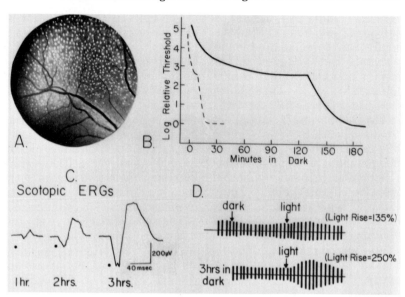

Figure 14.4   Fundus albipunctatus. A 38-year-old male with poor night vision all of his life. *A,* retina showing a multitude of small yellow white spots scattered throughout the retina but sparing the macular area. *B,* course of dark adaptation followed for a period of 3 hours. There is marked delay in *both* cone and rod adaptation. *C,* a normal scotopic ERG obtained only after a prolonged stay in the dark (3 hours). *D,* under normal testing conditions, markedly abnormal EOG light rise. After 3 hours in darkness, however, the *light rise/dark trough* ratio becomes normal.

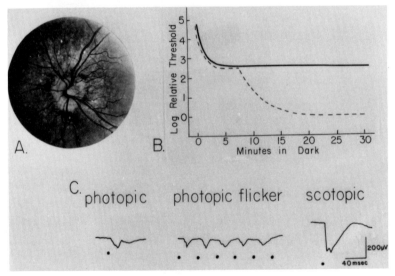

Figure 14.5   CSNB with nystagmus and myopia. The patient is a 22-year-old female who has had decreased acuity associated with nystagmus and poor night vision all her life. None of the signs or symptoms have changed over this period of time. *A,* fundus showing myopic disc changes, with the remainder of retina appearing normal. *B,* dark adaptation showing no evidence of rod participation when compared to the normal (*dashed line*). The cone system appears to adapt normally. *C,* ERG recordings under light- and dark-adapted conditions show only a negative a-wave (of normal amplitude) but no positive b-wave response.

bescens. However, unlike the latter disease, the visual fields and retinal arterioles are normal. The major diagnostic feature of this disease is the very slow adaptation properties of the cones and rods.[100] It can take longer than 1 hour for cones to obtain normal thresholds, and rod thresholds may be elevated for up to 2–3 hours before eventually attaining normal levels. Underlying this adaptometric abnormality is the prolonged regeneration time of cone and rod photopigments. All the visual functions measured subjectively or electrically return slowly to normal levels, going hand in hand with the prolonged return of photopigment concentration.

CSNB with myopia, nystagmus, and decreased visual acuity (Fig. 14.5) presents a major diagnostic problem. Not only is the patient nightblind, but the nystagmus and decreased vision, both present from birth, makes this disease appear at first glance similar to Leber's congenital amaurosis. However, the fundus, retinal arterioles, visual fields, cone thresholds, and EOG are all normal and serve to distinguish this disorder from a progressive generalized degeneration. This ERG is of the negative type (normal a-wave but absent b-wave), quite characteristic of the more common forms of CSNB.

15

Disorders of the Cone System

There has been some confusion with regard to nomenclature in this group of disorders. Despite a number of subcategories, they do, however, have in common a generalized loss in cone function, which results in the absence of an electroretinogram (ERG) flicker response. This diagnostic criterion excludes localized macular diseases which, though affecting a cone-rich area, do not markedly reduce the massed electrical responses of the entire cone population of the retina.

There exist the following broad categories of cone disorders:

Stationary: Rod monochromatism (complete and incomplete forms)
Cone monochromatism
Progressive: Cone dystrophy (hereditary or acquired)
Cone-rod dystrophy

Rod monochromatism (Fig. 15.1) is an autosomal recessive disease and is the most common and most visually debilitating form of the stationary congenital cone dysfunction syndromes. There are two forms of the disease, complete and incomplete, distinguishable primarily on the basis of the subjective findings. The absent ERG photopic response and the presence of normal rod function makes the diagnosis without difficulty. The pathogenetic abnormality is a congenital absence or near absence of cone receptors. Table 15.1 shows the main characteristics of the two types with the differences probably due to the number of functioning cones.

Cone Monochromatism. Achromatopsia (the complete lack of color discrimination) can also be produced if two of the three cone receptors are congenitally absent. Patients possessing only one of the three cone types (red, green, or blue) are called cone monochromats. Such patients cannot discriminate colors, since one cone type does not provide sufficient neural information to higher visual centers (see Appendix D).

However, the fact that the total cone population of the retina is intact, albeit with a single type cone, means that (1) the foveal architecture is preserved, (2) visual acuity is usually normal, though blue-cone monochromats are reported to have decreased acuity,[101] (3) flicker ERGs are normal (when done with white light or an appropriate color flash), (4) cone thresholds are normal if testing is done with appropriately colored stimuli, and (5) there is no nystagmus or photophobia.

The reader can get some idea of the workings of the visual system of a mono-cone monochromat by looking through a narrow band interference filter, with its peak transmission at 500 nm (blue-green). Every object looks blue-green, and it is not possible to make any hue discrimination at all. Being a trichromat, the observer know what "blue-green" is, but a cone monochromat has no spectral memory to which a color designation is referable.

Few clinicians will encounter this disorder. It is extremely rare (1 per 1,000,000)[102] and because of normal acuity such patients seldom are seen for eye care.

Those conditions known as *progressive cone dystrophies* require a more thorough examination for their elucidation than the stationary forms. Because they follow a degenerative course over a period of time, they are easily confused at various stages of their development with either a maculopathy or generalized tapetoretinal de-

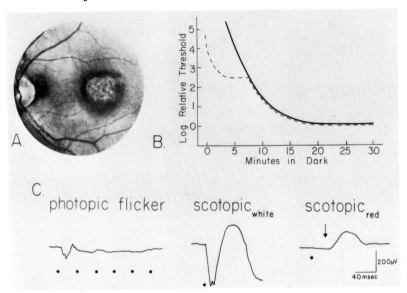

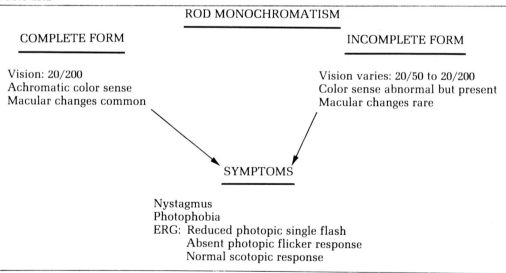

Figure 15.1 Rod monochromacy. A 51-year-old male had poor color vision with associated nystagmus and decreased vision all his life. Corrected visual acuity was 20/200 in each eye. *A*, both macular areas identical and showing granular pigmentation with loss of the pigment epithelium. The remainder of the fundus was normal. *B*, dark adaptation. The patient shows no evidence of cone function but a normal course of rod adaptation when compared to the normal (*dashed line*). *C*, no evidence of a flicker ERG response indicating generalized cone dysfunction. The scotopic response to white light is normal. Utilizing a red light test stimulus separates the ERG into cone and rod wavelets; the cone response is absent (*arrow*) in this patient, but there is a normal rod response.

Table 15.1

ROD MONOCHROMATISM	
COMPLETE FORM	INCOMPLETE FORM
Vision: 20/200 Achromatic color sense Macular changes common	Vision varies: 20/50 to 20/200 Color sense abnormal but present Macular changes rare

SYMPTOMS

Nystagmus
Photophobia
ERG: Reduced photopic single flash
        Absent photopic flicker response
        Normal scotopic response

generation. There are both hereditary and acquired forms of generalized progressive cone dystrophy, although the latter seems extremely rare.

Individuals with progresive cone dystrophy do not have any ocular problems at birth. The later signs are: progressive loss of vision, variable (unclassifiable) color vi-

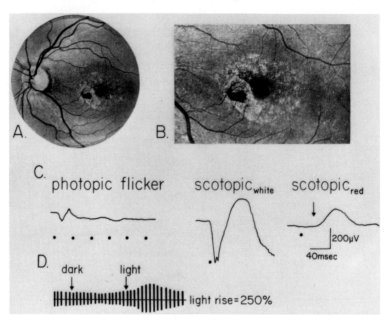

Figure 15.2 Progressive cone dysfunction (simplex). A 51-year-old male had normal vision until age 23. He noted a gradual loss of vision over a period of 5 years. Corrected visual acuity 20/200 OD and OS. *A*, macular area showing an irregular loss of pigment in a bullseye pattern. There is loss of the pigment epithelium in a ring surrounding the parafoveal area. *B*, details of the macular area. *C*, ERG showing no photopic flicker response. The scotopic response to white light, however, is normal. A red flash presented to the dark-adapted eye reveals no cone response (*arrows*), but a normal amplitude rod response. *D*, light rise of the electrooculogram is normal.

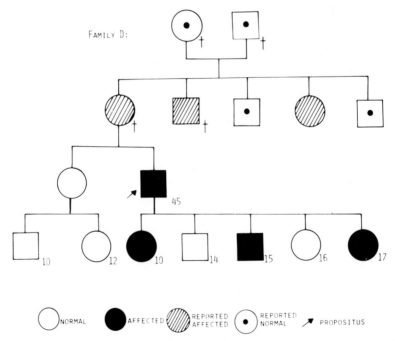

Figure 15.3 Progressive cone dysfunction. Pedigree demonstrating an autosomal dominant mode of inheritance in this family with late onset progressive cone dysfunction.

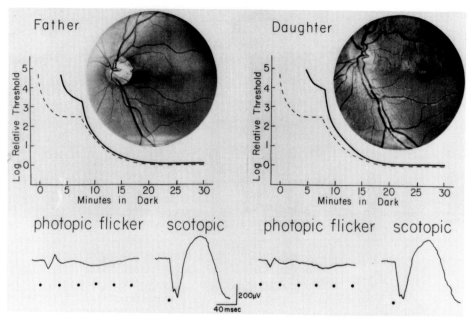

Figure 15.4 Progressive cone dysfunction (familial). The propositus is a 45-year-old male who had normal acuity until age 20 and then experienced a progressive loss of vision to 20/200 in each eye. He had five children, the oldest of which noted some decrease in vision for 2 years. He stated that his mother as well as a maternal uncle and aunt were affected with a condition similar to his. The figure represents the findings of the propositus and his 10-year-old daughter, who had no visual complaints. The retina of the father was normal, as was his daughter's. The dark adaptation curve of the father showed a marked abnormality in cone adaptation but normal rod adaptation. His ERG showed no flicker response but normal scotopic amplitudes. The daughter had a corrected visual acuity of 20/30 in each eye. The course of dark adaptation (tested in a peripheral region of the retina) shows a marked abnormality in cone function but normal rod recovery. The ERG showed no photopic flicker response but normal scotopic amplitudes. Her color vision was still normal due to the presence of still functioning foveal cones.

sion defects, macular changes, and photophobia. The ERG findings typically show a reduced photopic response to a single flash, an absent photopic flicker response, but normal scotopic amplitudes (Fig. 15.2). Such findings are reminiscent of rod monochromatism, but the late onset and deteriorating vision are prime distinguishing factors. In documented pedigrees, the mode of heritable transmission has been shown to be either autosomal dominant or autosomal recessive (Figs. 15.3 and 15.4).

To date, there is only one case report of *permanent, acquired, generalized cone dystrophy* following administration of a drug (furaltadone) to a 28-year-old patient with a systemic staphylococcus infection.[103] Interestingly, this patient retained a good deal of foveal function, as evidenced by her visual acuity (20/30) and relatively mild color loss. Again the predominating symptom of light dazzle and extinguished ERG flicker response signaled a generalized loss of cone function. Many drugs are known which affect color vision test results,[104] but rigorous criteria must be met before an *irreversible* generalized loss of cone function is established.

Finally, one must consider the possibility that a cone-rod dystrophy can occur as the end stage of a generalized late onset cone dystrophy. There may be little difference subjectively between the two conditions, and without functional testing performed over long intervals the distinction cannot be made.

16
Nystagmus and Decreased Vision from Birth

Every eye specialist will at some time be shown an infant with nystagmus who has not seen well since birth or shortly thereafter. In choosing among the several diseases which produce such symptoms, electrodiagnostic testing is of prime importance. Subjective tests are of no value because of the patient's age; objective measures of retinal function are therefore the only means by which a diagnosis may be made. It is often true that an adequate fundus evaluation is not possible with the child awake and moving. Ketamine anesthesia is of help, for it lasts sufficiently long to enable the examiner to do a complete fundus evaluation, refraction, electroretinogram (ERG), flash visual evoked potential (VEP), and ultrasound. Unlike most gas anesthetics, ketamine does not affect the ERG or VEP. It should be noted that full development of the ERG does not occur until approximately 2 months after full-term, and the VEP does not attain normal amplitudes for 1–2 years after birth. The ERG is the most important test in most instances; however, it should be delayed until retinal maturation has occurred. We feel most confident of our results if this test is done at age 6 months or later.

Table 16.1 lists several broad categories which should be considered when faced with the clinical assessment of an individual who has had poor vision and nystagmus from birth.

Disorders of the media are readily apparent, and the ERG will give objective evidence of the functioning of the retina. A flash VEP will likewise give some indication of foveal function, although the amplitudes will often be reduced. The presence of a normal ERG and VEP in association with normal ultrasound can give the physician a certain degree of confidence if surgical intervention is contemplated.

Optic nerve diseases can usually be diagnosed by ophthalmoscopic observation. However, small variations in the color, size, or shape of the optic nerve may be missed in an awake and moving child. This is especially true of optic nerve hypoplasia, where the commonly found ring of peripapillary atrophy may be mistaken for optic nerve and the true size of the nerve may not be appreciated.

In optic nerve disease (Fig. 16.1), the ERG to a flash stimulus will be normal, or occasionally the b-wave will be reduced in the presence of a normal a-wave. This latter change is assumed to derive from transsynaptic degeneration involving the bipolar cells, thus producing a b-wave reduction.[5]

Certain congenital or hereditary *macular diseases* may lead to nystagmus at birth. In addition, several *bilateral developmental diseases* of the entire retina, such as retrolental fibroplasia (RLF), and persistent hyperplastic primary vitreous (PHPV), where macular traction is usually noted causes similar signs and symptoms. The retinal dysplasia associated with 13-15 trisomy is also easily recognized with the ophthalmoscope, and the ancillary systemic findings will usually lead to the correct diagnosis. *Macular hypoplasia*, or more correctly from a pathogenetic viewpoint, lack of foveal differentiation, is seen in several diseases, the most common being in the various forms of albinism.[105]

94

Table 16.1
Causes Underlying Nystagmus and Decreased
Vision from Birth

I. Disorders of the media, e.g., corneal opacities and cataracts
II. Optic Nerve Diseases
   Coloboma
   Hypoplasia
   Atrophy
      Developmental
      Hereditary
III. Retinal Diseases
  A. Ophthalmoscopically Visible
     Macular Disease
      1. Colobomas (hereditary and infectious)
        Toxoplasmosis and inclusion cell disease
      2. Hypoplasia
        Albinism
        Aniridia
        Idiopathic
     Rare Bilateral Associations
     RLF, PHPV, retinal dysplasia
  B. Ophthalmoscopically Visible
     Leber's congenital amaurosis
     Rod monochromatism (achromatopsia)
     CSNB with nystagmus and decreased vision
IV. Congenital Nystagmus

While the classic "complete" oculocutaneous albino (tyrosinase-negative) with blond hair and skin, diaphanous irides, and lack of all fundus pigmentation is easily recognized, the tyrosinase-positive albino, in whom the skin may not be completely white, the irides may not be of normal color, and fundus pigmentation may be in the macula, can be more difficult to diagnose.[106] In a young child, examination under anesthesia will show the iris transillumination, the lack of peripheral fundus pigment, and an absence of any foveal landmarks. It is often useful to dilate one eye only so the fellow eye may be transilluminated in patients with suspected albinism.

The third type of albinism, ocular albinism, shows none of the skin changes but does show ocular changes similar to those of the tyrosinase-positive individual. Since this is an X-linked disorder, evaluation of the suspected female carrier may provide the diagnostic clues to make the diagnosis. Such a female will show spokewheel iris transillumination, as well as an unusual type of peripheral pigment granularity in the retina, although she herself shows neither nystagmus nor poor vision.[107]

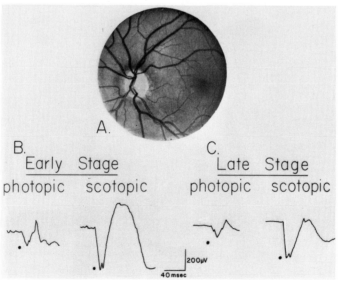

Figure 16.1 Optic atrophy. A 34-year-old female had been followed for 12 years after development of a craniopharyngioma. Visual acuity was reduced to light perception in the left eye. In the right eye there was a temporal field defect with normal vision. The left eye developed optic atrophy. An ERG, performed 1 year after diagnosis of the tumor, was normal. Twelve years later, the ERG showed reduced photopic b-waves. The scotopic response shows a large negative a-wave and a reduced b-wave.

All of the varieties of albinism will show normal ERGs. Indeed, the responses may be extremely large because of the light scatter in these lightly pigmented fundi.

The most difficult diagnoses in patients with poor vision and nystagmus from birth are noted in Table 16.1 as *ophthalmoscopically variable*. All have been discussed in previous chapters, but several points are worth reconsidering. In all of these diseases, the retina may appear normal, although in Leber's *congenital amaurosis*, retinal abnormalities are noted at some later stage. The ERG is absent since there is a widespread disorder of the RPE-photoreceptor complex akin to retinitis pigmentosa. In *rod monochromatism*, since there is a congenital absence of the cone receptors, the ERG will show a markedly abnormal or absent cone response, best seen with the flicker ERG, and a normal rod response. Patients with *CSNB* in which there is *associated nystagmus* are usually myopic but show a "negative" ERG with a deep a-wave and no b-wave.

Congenital nystagmus, a true entity, is really a diagnosis of exclusion after the other diseases have been ruled out. This particular group includes latent nystagmus and the autosomal dominant form of congenital nystagmus.

17
All Tests Considered

Having now considered the techniques and applications of all the commonly used electrical tests of visual function, there remains the task of indicating the situations in which a particular procedure yields the more definitive result. In this section we shall attempt to answer questions such as: Are there circumstances in which the electrooculogram (EOG) will prove more diagnostic than the electroretinogram (ERG)? Will a pattern-evoked visual evoked potential (VEP) provide the same information as a focal (foveal) ERG? Which test will unequivocally detect malingering? How important are oscillatory potentials? How does a bright flash ERG aid in presurgical evaluation of a retina obscured by cataract, corneal damage, or vitreous hemorrhage?

ERG *vs.* EOG

In the early EOG studies there was some suggestion that the light peak/dark trough change (Arden ratio) might be more diagnostic than the ERG in drug retinotoxicity and in early cases of generalized retinal degeneration.[75] An investigation designed specifically to compare EOG and ERG results for a variety of retinal diseases did not confirm this.[33] The EOG was also not shown to be more sensitive than the ERG in a large group of patients in different stages of chloroquine retinopathy.[108] Because the ERG and the EOG are tests predominantly of rod function, they tend to show similar trends. In generalized retinal disease, for example, both the b-wave amplitude and Arden ratio are diminished, with the degree of diminution dependent on the severity or stage of the disease.

For evaluating the many forms of congenital nyctalopia, the ERG is certainly the preferred test, since its wave-form changes are not only specific for each of the different types but also the wave configuration itself gives some clue as to the locus of the defect in the retina.

In the study of cone dysfunction syndromes, the ERG is the test of choice, since by adjusting the level of retinal adaptation and using repetitive flash stimuli the integrity of the entire cone population of the retina can be quickly assessed. Since the loss of large numbers of retinal cones do not affect the EOG light rise (rod monochromats have a normal Arden ratio), the EOG cannot be expected to be of much aid in distinguishing between the cone dysfunction syndromes.

THE EOG AND BEST'S DISEASE

There is one circumstance in which one would use the tedious and lengthy EOG recording rather than the faster, more flexible ERG. It is a curious fact that the EOG light rise is absent in patients with vitelliruptive macular dystrophy (Best's disease) while the ERG photopic and scotopic a- and b-waves in such patients are usually normal (Fig. 17.1). Even more significant is the finding that "carriers" of this moderately penetrant, dominantly inherited disease, who have no fundus changes, also show an abnormal EOG light rise.[109] Many studies have indicated that this abnormal EOG result is pathognomonic for Best's disease, as well as its rare variant known as butterfly dystrophy of the fovea.[110]

LOCAL (PATTERN) ERG *vs.* VEP

When the cone population of the fovea and perifoveal areas are specifically affected, as happens in most macular dis-

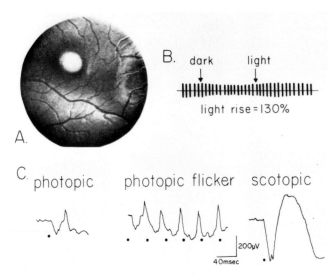

Figure 17.1 Vitelliruptive macular degeneration (Best's disease). The propositus was a 10-year-old Puerto Rican male who had no visual complaints and an acuity of 20/20 in each eye. A, in both macular areas, typical egg yolk lesions. B, reduced EOG light rise. C, ERG a- and b-waves for both photopic and scotopic recording conditions were normal.

eases, there will be a barely detectable change in the standard photopic flash or flicker ERG response. This occurs because only about 2% of the total cone population is located in the fovea, and this finding serves as a dramatic reminder of the great difference between a localized disturbance of a small cone-rich portion of the retina and a generalized dysfunction of the cone system. A local ERG, however, elicited with a reversing checkerboard or bar pattern covering a foveal-sized area (5°) is a direct measure of foveal integrity. The examiner is once again reminded that the average luminance of the pattern should not change during reversals (see Chapter 8). Since the peripheral retina is very sensitive to slight alterations in luminance fluctuations, the presence of such an artifact would seriously diminish the opportunities of recording from the foveal area itself. Even with an appropriate stimulus presentation, there is a great deal of difficulty in obtaining reliable recordings from naive subjects because of fixation wanderings and eye blinks.

It is these latter problems that may tempt the clinician to use the VEP, a more easily obtained potential which reflects predominantly foveal activity. Since the VEP derives from the visual cortex, however, an abnormality in the recorded waveform cannot point to a specific locus of disturbance in a particular portion of the visual system. Macular pathology, optic nerve disease, or cortical disturbance could each produce diminished VEP amplitudes. Ideally, a local ERG and VEP to the same pattern stimulus should be recorded simultaneously. The virtue of such a maneuver is that information about the fovea and postretinal portions of the visual pathway may be ascertained and compared.

Before leaving the topic of the pattern ERG, note must be taken of a recent ERG study which used pattern stimuli and showed that if the optic nerve of a cat was sectioned, the ERG response diminished and, after a few months, completely disappeared.[111] The flash ERG, however, remained the same amplitude as before optic nerve section. This surprising result can be interpreted in several ways, but the clinical implications (if confirmed in human studies) are quite clear. At least some portion of the recordable ERG is sensitive to the spatial distribution of light; whether it is the ganglion cells themselves or other structures in the inner plexiform layer[112] is not specifically known. Such results might also explain why pattern ERGs are decreased in amblyopic patients.[23]

DETECTION OF MALINGERING AND CONFIRMATION OF VISUAL LOSS

The VEP is the best objective procedure of choice for evaluating patients with suspected hysterical loss of vision or who are consciously malingering. The examiner should keep in mind that, for this purpose, flash stimuli are not as useful as highly textured pattern stimuli, although both may play a role.

For example, if a patient claims to have severely reduced vision (hand movements or light perception) in one eye and normal acuity in the fellow eye, one would expect a markedly reduced flash VEP response in the affected eye. A normal response in this eye would confirm a diagnosis of malingering. However, if patients complain of more subtle loss of vision (20/40 to 20/200) or if the vision is bilaterally affected to an equal degree, VEP testing should be conducted with pattern stimuli at decreasing spatial frequency and contrast.

Since a reversing checkerboard pattern, generated on a TV screen, can be manipulated with respect to check size, contrast, and alternation rate, judicious control of these variables allows study of visual acuity, as well as generation of contrast sensitivity function in a completely objective manner (Chapter 10). However, there is one exception to this approach to visual testing. A patient with a lesion in visual association area 18 will be blind as judged by any behavioral test, yet the VEP (the origin of which is derived from the *lower* visual area 17 can be normal).[113] The final caveat of VEP testing is clear: if any doubt remains as to the nature of the loss of vision, a neurologic evaluation should be recommended.

Table 17.1 provides a summary of the results from several tests of electrical function which the clinician can use to quickly

find the one which would be the most relevant for a specific type of visual abnormality.

OSCILLATORY POTENTIALS AND THEIR PRESUMED CLINICAL USE

It is quite simple, without any additional electronic gear, to reveal the several wavelets—the oscillatory potentials—which ride on the ERG b-wave. High intensity flashes at 1-minute intervals presented to the dark-adapted eye are the most efficient conditions for eliciting these potentials.[114] However, even under the best stimulus arrangements, the large, slowly developing b-wave masks the underlying oscillations. If a study of these potentials is of importance, the clinician need only increase the low band-pass frequency setting on the preamplifier, which will emphasize the faster components while sacrificing the slower ones (Appendix A, section II). Figure 17.2 shows the effect of increasing the low frequency band-pass to 60 Hz (the high frequency cut is left at the usual setting of about 300 Hz). The b-wave is absent, and several oscillatory potentials are clearly visible. If the entire ERG is small, then averaging techniques will have to be used to see the smaller oscillations.

Under what circumstances would the clinician want to observe oscillatory potentials? Some years ago, Yonemura et al.[115] obtained results which indicated that in the early stages of diabetic retinopathy and in some instances before diabetic retinal changes were noted, there was a diminution of oscillatory potential amplitude. However, Gjötterberg[116] could not confirm these results. More recently, Yonemura[117] has reinvestigated the relation between oscillatory potentials and diabetes and now claims that the latency of the potentials is increased in patients with early stages of retinopathy. In the course of our own studies, we have measured the latency of these potentials in many patients representing various grades of diabetic retinopathy and have not been able to detect an increased time to peak of these responses.

In his early studies Yonemura[115] also

Table 17.1
Use of the Various Electrical Tests in the Diagnosis of Visual Loss

	Standard ERG	EOG light rise	Pattern ERG	VEP[b]
Macular disease	Normal	Normal[a]	Reduced	Abnormal
Optic nerve disease	Normal	Normal	May be abnormal	Abnormal
Higher center disease	Normal	Normal	Normal	Abnormal
Hysteria or malingering	Normal	Normal	Normal	Normal
Generalized tapetoretinal degeneration	Abnormal	Abnormal	Abnormal	Abnormal

[a] In vitelliform dystrophy of the macula (Best's disease) and butterfly dystrophy of the macula, this test is usually abnormal.
[b] Abnormality may be either a reduction in amplitude (as in early macular disease), or an increase in latency (as in some forms of optic nerve disease).

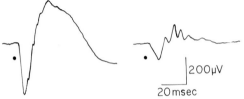

Figure 17.2   To unmask the oscillatory potentials riding the ascending limb of the ERG b-wave, raise the low frequency band-pass filter of the preamplifier to about 60 Hz. This will effectively remove all the slower ERG components, including the large b-wave, and only the fast frequency components remain (compare the filtered ERG (*right*) with the normally recorded trace (*left*)). To achieve large amplitude oscillatory potentials, a pair of high intensity flashes are presented to the dark-adapted eye with an interval of 1 minute separating them; a record is made of the second response.

reported that gross retinal pathology produced by vascular disease, retinal detachment, and macular degeneration may be associated with decreased oscillatory potential amplitudes. While this certainly seems to be true, the ophthalmoscope is likely to be a more valuable aid to diagnosis than the disappearance of oscillatory potentials.

Only recently, has the origin of the oscillatory potentials in the vertebrate retina been investigated with the same zeal as other ERG components. Earlier work suggested the amacrine cells as their origin.[118] At present, the oscillatory potentials, like the clinicially recorded b-wave, probably result from the complex interaction between the amacrines, the newly discovered interplexiform cells,[119] and perhaps the ubiquitous Müller cells. When the uncertainty about their origin is resolved in the laboratory, then the diagnostic role of the clinically recorded oscillatory potentials will be on more secure ground.

RETINAL EVALUATION WHEN THE FUNDUS IS OBSCURED

In assessing retinal function in diseases where the retina is not visible, certain considerations must be kept in mind. First, the ERG, being a mass response, is unable to assess the function of specific retinal areas. Thus, a normal ERG may be present with severe macular disease and, conversely, the ERG may be absent even with a functional macular region (e.g., retinitis pigmentosa). Second, very dense hemorrhage may prevent any significant amount of light from reaching the retina. With these admonitions in mind, a logical approach to the use of electrodiagnostic tests in opaque media can be formulated.

Corneal and lenticular opacities lend themselves nicely to ERG recording since such abnormalities act as light diffusers and do not themselves obscure ERG evaluation. Using the ERG to assess retinal function following a vitreous hemorrhage is somewhat more difficult. Fuller et al.[120] have established a protocol for the use of the "bright-flash" ERG in such patients. The rationale for using a high intensity light is to provide a sufficient stimulus to infer the presence or absence of viable retina.

Several points should be noted, however, which can guide the clinician in his use of this test as a means of determining retinal function. First, if an ERG is recordable, it would indicate that most of the retina is intact, but does not demonstrate the extent of macular function and what the ultimate visual outcome might be following removal of the hemorrhage. Second, if the ERG is not recordable, it may mean that most of the retina is damaged. However, such a finding does not indicate whether the macular area may be functional, and likewise does not reveal whether the hemorrhage may have been so dense as to preclude any light from reaching the retina. In such cases it has recently been shown that removal of dense vitreous hemorrhage in the presence of an absent ERG may reveal large areas of functional retina.[121]

Several approaches have been designed to assure maximal light input to the retina in doing "bright flash" ERG testing. Increasing the lamp output by using a longer duration flash (in the millisecond range) such as is common in photography has proved quite successful.[120] One problem should be mentioned with regard to this bright flash technique. When a high capacitance flash tube is held close to the eye, the chances for photoelectric artifact generation are enhanced. For this reason the lamp casing may have to be shielded

with metal plate (see also Appendix A, section IV). Before investing in another piece of apparatus, the clinician should first attempt to increase the flash brightness by simply placing the Grass photostimulator just a few inches from the eye.

Also of possible use in such cases may be the "flash" VEP, especially if a normal fellow eye is present. If the VEP in the affected eye is similar to that of the normal eye, then one may assume that both the macular area, as well as the optic nerve, are normal. Normalcy of this response in conjunction with a recordable ERG would give a great deal of assurance to the physician that successful surgery will find a functional retina. Horwitz et al.[122] have recently utilized a fiber optic bundle to deliver light transsclerally so as to evoke both an ERG and VEP response. Tenon's capsule is dissected away on the temoral side of the globe, and the eye is rotated to expose the scleral aspect of the fovea. A fiber optic bundle is applied to a point on the sclera approximating the fovea, and a transscleral VEP is recorded. This ingenious technique provides invaluable presurgical information about foveal integrity, and when circumstances demand, it is a novel adjunct to more standard procedures.

While electrodiagnostic tests in themselves are not absolute in patient assessment, their use, along with ultrasonography, as well as a knowledge of the disease process which caused the insult (e.g., diabetes, trauma, blood dyscrasias), can provide additional information for better surgical guidance.

Appendix A

ERG: Technical Data

I. SHIELDING AND FILTERING REQUIREMENTS

Because of the high gain requirements of the electroretinogram (ERG) (minimally 100 μV/cm), the presence of 60 Hz mains hum with amplitudes exceeding 20μV will seriously interfere with trace fidelity. Mains hum is present as an in-phase signal at both the recording and indifferent (reference) electrodes. Differential amplification, which is usually used in biomedical work, reduces such common mode signals and selectively operates on the out-of-phase ERG signal. Fortunately, the high common mode rejection ratios (100,000:1 is typical) in modern amplifiers will usually eliminate all but the most pervasive 60 Hz background noise.

In any case, the clinician has to be prepared to deal effectively with a "noisy" trace. First, be sure that it is actually 60 Hz interference that is the interfering component of the recording. Examine the trace at a fast paper speed or faster-than-normal scope sweep. A 60-Hz signal has a regular sinusoidal appearance which is superimposed on the tracing. Figure A.1 shows how "spreading out" the trace on a scope can uncover and identify the noise.

It is important also to distinguish the regular 60-Hz artifact from other types of interference. Infrequently, high voltage TV signals or stray transient electric fields from elevator motors may be picked up. The latter type of interference may be filtered out effectively but usually requires consultation with an electronics engineer. Most often, the clinician may notice irregular bursts of interference on the recording of the type shown in Figure A.2.

Fast bursts of noise are usually due to muscle spasms such as those induced by jaw tightening or forehead wrinkling. In addition, a strong blink reflex or eye movement may saturate the amplifiers in a positive or negative direction, completely blocking the flow of current, thus preventing the display of any output. A flat line will appear under such circumstances. Finally, ubiquitous blink reflexes will produce annoying trace deflections. Blinks may be easily distinguished from ERGs which they resemble, because they occur *in the absence* of a flash, reminding us again of the absolute need for a stimulus artifact on the record. No miracle of electronics can substitute for a relaxed, cooperative, patient. Reliable ERG interpretation clearly requires the clinician to be aware of, and recognize, all the different types of recording artifacts.

Since the electrical environments vary widely from location to location, the clinician should be sceptical of manufacturing claims of "low noise" levels for their instruments. Have the device demonstrated in the area in which the ERG is actually going to be performed—before purchase. Be sure that the salesman is aware that you do not want to record the ERG with a "passive" 60-Hz filter slipped into place. More about this point in a later section. Many types of recording equipment will require copper screen shielding around the patient to eliminate 60-Hz interference. Before one considers this awkward, expensive solution, however, all other possibilities should first be considered. Here are a few recording tips designed to reduce whatever mains hum may be present in any recording location:

1. Keep all electrode leads as short as possible. Excessively long leads act like pickup antennae for superfluous signals.
2. Recheck the electrode attachments. Particularly note whether the forehead disc is firmly adherent to the skin, and contains an appropriate amount of electrode jelly.

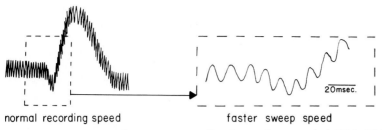

normal recording speed   faster sweep speed

Figure A.1 Mains hum (60 Hz), when present, will ride on the recorded ERG. This particular source of interference can be identified by increasing the sweep speed of the scope or polygraph. A sinusoidal wave-form with a duty cycle of about 17 msec will be easily seen.

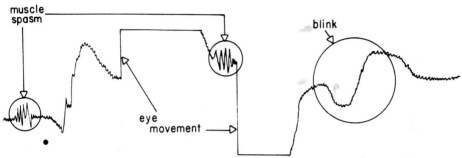

Figure A.2 Some typical artifacts which may be seen on ERG records are shown in this extended tracing. Fast bursts of muscle spasm deriving from jaw or forehead muscle activity are common, as well as large shifts of base line which most commonly occur when the patient shifts his eye or attempts a blink. Blink artifacts, which often resemble ERG responses, can be separated from retinal electrical activity, because they occur in the absence of a flash stimulus.

3. Adding an extra drop of artificial tears to the contact lens electrode while it is in the patient's eye will reduce the resistance and improve a noisy signal.
4. If recordings have been adequate for some time and then suddenly deteriorate, check the electrode pin connections first. Often, the fine leads break off, or fray badly inside the insulation and make poor connection to the terminal pin connector. Wires also tend to disconnect on the contact lens end of the lead and should be carefully checked with a magnifying glass. Such faults can be quickly tracked down with an ohmmeter. An infinite or very high resistance reading (in excess of 100 kohms) indicates a broken connection. In any case, change to a different contact lens electrode or reference disc to assure yourself on this point. Before pulling any leads out of the input terminal, however, check to see that they were correctly inserted to begin with!

II. AMPLIFIER SETTINGS AND ERG CALIBRATION PROCEDURES

The ERG wave-forms have a finite duration. Measured from the flash, photopic ERGs are over in about 50 msec and scotopic waves in about 100 to 200 msec—fortunately, just a bit faster than the blink reflex. The ERG does contain as a major fast transient, the a-wave, but in clinical recording situations, no very slowly changing potentials (such as the c-wave) are usually determined. Therefore, as a rule, the low and high band-pass frequency settings on the amplifiers may be set at about 1 and 300 Hz, respectively. This will allow reasonable fidelity of waves having components, the periods of which range from as long as 1 sec to as short as 3 msec. Polygraphs cannot faithfully reproduce signals varying faster than 50 Hz so that the high frequency attenuation is an intrinsic limitation in such instruments.

There is often an understandable degree of panic when confronting the complex instrumentation of the modern polygraph or oscilloscope for the first time. Many individuals simply find out what settings other workers use, imitate them exactly, and do every ERG or EOG in a rote manner. The following section, therefore, is designed to take some of the mystery out of the large assemblage of dials with which the clinician should be familiar. If nothing else, it will provide the interested ERG worker with enough background to ask intelligent questions of overzealous purveyors of electronic equipment or to seek advice from electronic engineers when problems concerning ERG wave-form characteristics arise.

Even the most cursory examination of ERG records show them to be composed of fast and slow components. The development of the a-wave, as well as the rising portion of the photopic b-wave, are represented by rapid changes in voltage. A dim flash in the dark, on the other hand, produces a slow-rising (scotopic) b-wave. The low and high frequency attenuation dials simply limit, by changing resistor and capacitor values, the responsiveness of the amplifier to these developing waves. Therefore, the frequency characteristics of an amplifier should be such as to allow visualization of the fast components, as well as to allow complete representation of the slower ones, e.g., the large scotopic b-waves.

It is unfortunately a fact of life that most off-the-shelf electronic recording instruments are not designed for a specific purpose. Polygraphs and oscilloscopes are constructed to fulfill the needs of many specialized disciplines. The user must, therefore, learn which settings on the dial apply to his immediate application which is, in the present case, the faithful recording of an ERG trace. The clinician must know *how fast* some of the components develop and *how long*, under ideal conditions, they maintain themselves before returning to the base line of their own accord. From laboratory records of ERGs we can specify some of this needed waveform information. The very fast components are represented by the developing a-wave and rising portion of the b-wave which reach their troughs and peaks in a few milliseconds. As already mentioned, high frequency filter attenuation settings should be such as to allow reproduction of

waves which repeat every 1/0.003 seconds or 333 Hz. That is why, when possible, the high frequency attenuation setting is placed at 300 to 1000 Hz for scope recording. Remember that although polygraph recordings are limited on the high frequency end by pen inertia, they do provide reasonable reconstructions of a- and b-wave potentials. Low frequency settings for scope and polygraph display require a bit more consideration.

Ideally, one would like to have *no* attenuation of the low frequency components (i.e., DC recording) and thus be able to accurately record, for example, not only full b-wave amplitudes but also perhaps even the elusive c-wave, which originates in the pigment epithelium and occurs one-half second or more *after* the flash. Two factors weigh against using DC recording. First, *any* eye movement will be reflected as a huge base line shift which may take many seconds to restore to the original level on the center of the scope screen or middle of the paper strip. Such base line shifts often take the trace off the scope display or override the pen excursion on the polygraph, during which time no recording may take place. For clinical purposes, therefore, we must compromise the low frequency reproduction of the ERG. The question then becomes—by how much?

It will soon become clear that although we can increase the low frequency attenuation to a point where the base line will be quite stable—hardly shifting with eye movements—the development of the b-wave will be seriously impaired. This is illustrated in Figure A.3, which shows the effect of increasing the low frequency attenuation from values which allow passage of very slowly changing potentials, i.e., 0.1 Hz, to a much higher cut-off value of 60 Hz. Note the effect, particularly on the b-wave amplitude. Obviously, one could work comfortably with a low frequency setting of about 10 Hz which, as will be shown later, will attenuate waveforms having a duration of 100 msec by about 30%. Since the time occupied by the developing b-wave, as measured from the trough of the a-wave to where it reaches

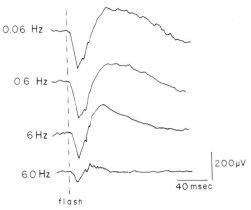

0.06 Hz

0.6 Hz

6 Hz

60 Hz

200 μV

40 msec

flash

Figure A.3   Effect of changing the low band-pass filter setting on the ERG preamplifier. In the sequence of tracings shown, the high band-pass is maintained at 300 Hz, and the low band-pass frequency setting is raised in decade steps from 0.06 to 60 Hz. Note the marked reduction in amplitude and wave shape characteristics of the ERG a- and b-waves recorded with low band-pass frequencies of 0.6 Hz or higher.

the base line is rarely more than 60 msec, this is a reasonable low frequency setting. In practice, however, a frequency of about 1 or 2 Hz is usually used as the low frequency band-pass.

While many instruments (particularly oscilloscopes) provide clearly designated values of low and high frequency settings, others may not. How then do you know whether a particular apparatus provides appropriate band-pass characteristics with which to record an ERG?

With the aid of a square wave calibrator such as the Grass SWC-1B, all the necessary frequency prerequisites of a recording system can be delineated. The calibrator is applied across the three inputs of the ERG terminal box so that the (+), (−), and ground pins of the calibrator are inserted into the contact lens, reference, and ground receptacles, respectively. The device can generate square waves with a variety of micro- and millivolt amplitudes at several repetition rates on the scope screen or polygraph paper. It also produces a square wave which will maintain itself at a given voltage value as long as the "manual" button is pressed. For example, Figure A.4 shows the generation of a 100-μV square wave on a polygraph. As the figure indicates, the button is depressed until the trace returns to the base line, and then it is released. It should be noted that

many polygraphs have built-in square wave calibration signals of 50-μV amplitude. Check your polygraph manual! If the paper speed is run at the usual speed of 50 mm/sec, each mm represents 20 msec of time (1/50 = 0.02 sec). Since band-pass settings are actually produced by a combination of resistors and capacitors inside the amplifier, the top of the square wave is transformed, as shown in the figure, into an exponential function. By convention, the time constant of this exponential is represented by the time elapsed for the function to drop to 37% of its peak value. In the example shown, this is the time for the trace to fall from the peak of 100 μV down to 37μV, which is measured out on the recording paper to be 5 mm or 100 msec (5 mm x 20 msec/mm). The intersection indicated by the *dashed lines* and *arrow* occurs at 100 msec, which denotes the duration of the time constant, often expressed as T or RC (Resistance × Capacitance).

All AC coupled amplifiers lose sensitivity at extremely low frequency signals. The so-called turnover frequency point represents the frequency at which the sensitivity is reduced a specific amount—usually 30%, sometimes given as 3 decibels 'down' or −3 db. The time constant is simply related to the turnover frequency (F) for the 3-db loss in sensitivity by the

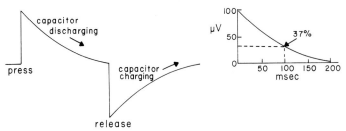

Figure A.4   Calibrating the amplitude and time course characteristics of an ERG recording. A single 100-μV square wave signal is applied to the inputs of the amplifier by pressing the button of a pulse generator, waiting until the signal reaches the base line, and then releasing the button. The time it takes for the signal to fall to 37% of its maximum voltage (here shown to be 100 msec) is the time constant for the system. The amplification of the system is verified by noting how many divisions are encompassed by the 100-μV peak voltage.

following relation: $F = \dfrac{1}{2\pi T}$. In the example, where $T = 0.1$ sec (100 msec): $\dfrac{1}{(2\pi \cdot 0.1)}$

= 1.6 Hz. (The low frequency attenuation dial settings on the better scopes such as the Tektronix are actually the −3 db turnover frequency points.) However, it is the 100-msec time constant value that is more relevant than the turnover frequency. For full development, the b-wave requires about 60 to 70 msec, therefore, a time constant as long as 100 msec assures you that little attenuation of such waves will occur.

Many widely used polygraphs do not specify low frequency attenuation settings as such. Rather, there are dials marked "half-amplitude frequency attenuation" and associated time-constant indications. A half-amplitude frequency setting indicates the turnover frequency which is attenuated by one-half (sometimes noted as the 6-db frequency). You certainly do not want the b-wave amplitude reduced by this amount, so the half-amplitude setting is set at 0.3 or 1 Hz (giving time constants of 0.24 and 0.1 sec, respectively—quite long enough for good b-wave reproduction).

The gain (sensitivity) of the system can also be checked with the same procedure shown in Figure A.4. For example, the 100-μV square wave measures out 1 cm on the recording paper or on the oscilloscope screen. Each mm is, therefore, equivalent to 10μV. The amplitude of any ERG component subsequently recorded can now be simply calculated. For example, a b-wave

measuring a height of 15 mm on the recording is 10 x 15 equaling 150 μV in amplitude.

A good rule of thumb is to try to work with a low frequency attenuation setting at least twice as long as the frequency of the wave to be viewed. The b-wave, for example, has a duration of about 60 msec (0.06 sec) and crudely represents a wave of 17 Hz so a low frequency setting which passes a wave of half that frequency (twice as long) or about 9 Hz *without* amplitude attenuation is adequate. Similarly, a high frequency setting should be such as to pass waves executing oscillations *twice the required frequency.* If the leading edges of the a- and b-waves reach peaks in about 5 msec (0.005 sec), then a high frequency attenuation setting of 2(1/0.005) equaling 400 Hz would be appropriate.

The paper speed of a polygraph or sweep speed of an oscilloscope can likewise be verified by running square waves of known duration and frequency into the input terminals. For example, the output of a calibrator set to give a 200-msec duration wave at a 5/sec repetition rate is fed into the polygraph. (Most calibrators output square waves having an equal duty cycle, so that a 5-cps signal will automatically yield a 200-msec long positive deflection followed by a 200-msec "off" duration. Similarly, a 10-Hz signal has equal 100-msec on-off deflections.) Check that your calibrator has equal on-off times irrespective of frequency before proceeding. If the paper speed is correct, then each wave will measure exactly 10 mm (since at 50 mm/

sec, each mm = 20 msec); the interval between waves will also be 10 mm, and there will be exactly 3 square waves reproduced for each 50 mm length of recording paper.

Likewise, a 50-Hz square wave should produce polarity changes every large division width on an oscilloscope when the horizontal sweep speed is set at 20 msec/division.

III. STROBE FLASH CALIBRATION

For clinical purposes, the manufacturer's statement about duration and power for the lamp are satisfactory. As mentioned previously it is probably more pertinent to have a set of average normal ERG responses against which to compare affected patients than to know in photometric terms exactly how bright the flash is. Provided that flash-to-eye distance is kept constant, the pupils are dilated, and the ocular media is clear, such comparisons will always have a high degree of internal validity. However, if ERGs from different clinics are to be studied, a more rigorous intensity calibration is required.

1. Energy Calibration of Intensity. Some version of a thermopile is used for energy measure of flash output. Typically, these instruments absorb the quanta on a sensitized surface during the brief flash and convert the heat generated by the absorption into a small voltage. The thermopile is calibrated in watts per volt (more realistically $\mu W/\mu V$). However, much of the energy output of the flash either does not reach the retina (such as the ultraviolet) or is not absorbed by the visual pigments (such as the infrared); hence, unless one goes through an elaborate spectral matching maneuver, the energy calibration is not "visually" relevant.

2. Photometric Calibration of the Flash. While measuring filament types of light sources is a straightforward matter, the brief duration of the strobe flash precludes the use of most light-measuring devices. However, a quite simple procedure is available to the clinician which does not involve elaborate instrumentation. If the strobe lamp can be made to appear as a steady luminance instead of a flash of short duration, a subjective "null"-type photometer such as the Ilford S.E.I. can be used to measure the brightness of this "steady" light. To accomplish this, the strobe is made to flash repetitively at a rate above the flicker fusion threshold. If the lamp cannot be driven above 30 flashes/sec it still may be made to appear steady at lower repetition rates by holding a neutral density filter in front of the photometer head. Following is a typical example of such a luminance calibration.

A strobe flash repeating at 30 Hz appears as "steady" when viewed through a 2.0 log density filter held in front of the measuring head of the S.E.I. photometer. The null-point match reading of the photometer is log 1.5 foot lamberts. Converting foot lamberts (ft. L) to the more commonly used millilambert (mL) luminance units, multiply by 1.047 (1.5 log ft. L = 31.6 ft. L. × 1.047 = 33.1 mL). Obviously, the measured luminance is not steady, and some compensation must be made for this fact. For example, if the flash was on half the time and off half the time but looked steady, the measured luminance would represent only half the value of the true luminance.

The duration of the strobe lamp can be directly measured using a photodiode outputting to a scope display, or by assuming that the manufacturer's specification is correct. Most strobes such as the Grass PS 22 have durations ranging between 10 and 20 μsec, depending on the intensity setting. For our example, we will choose a 20-μsec duration. During a 1-sec interval the flash is "on" 30 times, each flash occupying 1/20 millionths of a second! Therefore, the total time the 30 flashes occupy is only 30 × 20 μsec, equaling 600 μsec or 0.0006 sec. The measured luminance must, therefore, be multiplied by 1/0.0006 or 1667 to compensate for the 'off' periods since these "off" periods are clearly much longer than the total "on time" of brief flashes. The final calculation is then to multiply the measured luminance of 33.1 mL by the weighting factor 1667, which gives 55,177 mL or 4.742 log mL. Final adjustment is now made for the 2.0 log density filter through which the strobe flashes were originally measured, i.e., 4.742 + 2.0 = 6.742 log mL. Millilambert values may be converted to candela/m² or trolands using tables found in many sourcebooks, such as Le Grand's.[123]

IV. CHANGING FLASH-TO-EYE DISTANCE AND BRIGHT FLASH TECHNIQUES

Under most circumstances the clinician wants to maintain a constant flash-to-eye distance for standardization purposes. This distance is usually 12 to 18 inches if a ganzfeld is not used. However, it is the resulting ERG wave-form that will often indicate that an adjustment in flash distance should be made. If, for example, the low intensity flash setting produces a prominent a-wave in the dark-adapted eye, the flash is probably too close. Low intensity scotopic stimuli should produce an ERG composed essentially of only a b-wave, with perhaps a very small (less than 20 μV) a-wave notch. In ganzfeld stimulation, where distance is not a factor, only the ERG wave-form gives a clue to the flash intensity.

Nevertheless, there are some ocular diseases which prevent adequate amounts of light from reaching the retina. In these instances it may be necessary to forget standard practices and move the flash lamp quite close to the eye. Halving the flash distance, for example, will double the amount of energy falling on the retina and greatly enhance the chances of quanta penetrating hemorrhage or other vitreal obstructions. Usually, all one wants to know in these situations is whether or not viable retina lies beneath the opaque material. This sort of information, crude as it is, may prove invaluable prior to vitrectomy or traumatic cataract surgery. A longer duration, high intensity flash such as the sort used in photography can be substituted for the brief duration strobes usually used in ERG work. In this procedure, a photodiode stimulated by the flash may be used to provide an artifact on the polygraph or scope trace. Alternately, the strobe and scope may be triggered externally with an appropriate stimulus pulse generator. Such photo strobe lamps, however, produce large photoartifacts by virtue of their huge capacitative discharge. This artifact will appear directly on the ERG trace, and will often be larger than the ERG itself! The problem with using such "bright flash" intensities then becomes one of eliminating the photoartifact.[124] The following section provides some techniques to distinguish between

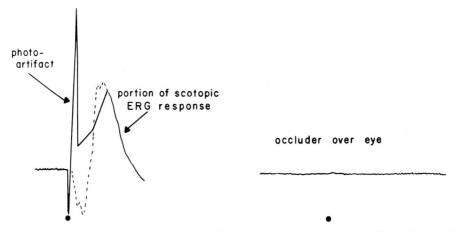

Figure A.5 The action of light on the exposed metal parts of a contact lens electrode or reference electrode can produce a photoartifact large enough to mask the ERG. To verify that the artifact is photically generated, occlude the face of the patient from the flash, and repeat the recording (*right tracing*). If the artifact is still present, then it is of electrical origin, probably deriving from the capacitor discharge of the flash apparatus.

the two major forms of artifact which may arise—electrical and photic.

V. EVALUATING PHOTO- AND FLASH ARTIFACTS

The effect of intense light on metal surfaces can produce potentials at least as large as the ERG itself. Since photoartifacts occur simultaneously with the flash, they will, unlike an eye blink or muscle noise, be easily confused with retinal response. However, unlike the ERG, they will occur with no detectable latency and be of short duration, as shown in Figure A.5. If the eye and active electrode and reference electrode are occluded by a piece of cardboard (leaving the flash in place), no ERG *or artifact* will be present if the latter was photically generated. If the artifact *does not* disappear when the active eye electrode and *reference electrode* are occluded, then the artifact is electrical and probably derives from electrical capacitance produced by the flash apparatus.

Check the type of contact lens electrode you are using. Often a photoartifact is produced by the commonly used bipolar lens electrode (in which a silver-coated speculum serves as reference). This may be eliminated by changing to a forehead reference.

Electrical artifacts can usually be eliminated by constructing a small cage of copper wire screening around the flash lamp and grounding the screen. Keeping the electrode leads short and twisting the active and inactive leads around each other will also help.

Finally, a very fine, fast, spike artifact on the ERG trace is sometimes seen on scope recording (but rarely on polygraphs).

Such artifacts will not interfere with the visualization of the response. Indeed, artifacts having such a configuration will prove useful, accurate markers for latency measurements.

VI. THE USE OF ACTIVE 60 HZ FILTERS

Passive notch filters labelled "line" filters are often provided on preamplifiers. While eliminating the 60-Hz main noise, they also wreak havoc with the fast components of the ERG—the a-wave and rising portion of the b-wave. Figure A.3 shows the effect of recording an ERG with various electrical filters in place. The 60-Hz filter corresponds to a "line" filter. Note particularly the attenuation of the a- and b-waves.

Tunable "notch" filters exist which do not compromise the amplitude of the major ERG components, e.g., the a- and b-waves. However, there are two sorts of electronic distortion these devices introduce which may seriously affect other ERG characteristics, namely, latency and a certain degree of attenuation of frequencies below and above the 60-Hz point. If latency measures or oscillatory potential evaluations are made with a 60-Hz active notch filter in place, take the following precautions. First, determine exactly how much phase shifting and attenuation occurs at frequencies analogous to a- and b-wave development times, i.e., about 100 Hz and, second, examine the filter at those frequencies characteristic of the oscillatory potentials. Check the specification sheets provided with active filters *before purchase.*

Appendix B
EOG: Technical Data

For electrooculography (EOG), which requires recording of slow saccades, the half amplitude setting of a polygraph or scope should be set at about 0.1 cycles Hz (i.e., time constant about 1.0 sec). As mentioned before, high frequency settings above 50 Hz are superfluous on polygraphs because of the great inertia of the recording pens. Frequency settings higher than 50 Hz are certainly indicated on the driver amplifier modules of the Grass instrument, but they relate *only to the internal amplification characteristics*, not to the actual ink writing display.

The band-pass frequency settings on the amplifier should be wide enough to ensure faithful reproduction of the saccade. For a slowly developing eye movement potential such as that obtained with the sinusoidal stimulator, a low pass of about 1 Hz is required. Since there are no high frequency components of diagnostic significance in this wave-form, the upper band pass limit can be set to 30 Hz. For the ballistic saccade movements produced by two isolated fixation lights, the low frequency can be set up to 2 to 5 Hz, but the high frequency attenuation must be raised to at least 100 Hz so that the amplitude of the saccade (which occurs as a fast transient, as in the *inset* of Fig. 4.4) is not diminished. The noise problems (mainly from mains voltage) are not as severe as those encountered in ERG work since the gain required for EOG recording is usually 2 to 5 times less. Obviously, a 60-Hz "notch filter" should be avoided while recording

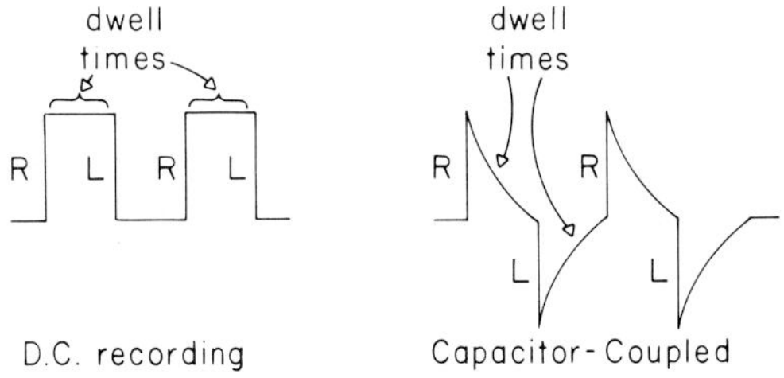

Figure B.1 Although DC recording will faithfully preserve the wave-form characteristics of EOG saccades and the associated dwell times, it is overly sensitive to changes of skin resistance and eye blinks. Using the more stable, capacitor-coupled type of amplification with a low frequency band-pass of about 1 Hz permits accurate recording of the *right* and *left* eye swings which are the only properties of the recording used to measure the light-induced EOG changes.

ballistic saccades since it will seriously distort the EOG trace.

Direct current (DC) recording of the EOG accurately reproduces the ballistic saccade but has serious drawbacks. Even small changes in skin resistance, for example, will produce a drifting pen movement which precludes continuous recordings of EOG responses. Since the wave-form characteristics of the EOG are of no diagnostic importance in determining the light rise, DC amplification is unnecessary.

Figure B.1 illustrates the difference in appearance between a DC-recorded EOG and one recorded with a low band-pass filter in place. Only the eye dwell time is not reproduced accurately with capacitor-coupled amplification.

Appendix C
Patient Safety Considerations

The electrical hazards most commonly encountered in electroretinograms (ERGs) or other biological recordings derive from accidental passage of mains current through the various electrodes attached to the patient. It is now generally recognized that minute electric currents, much smaller than will produce a sensation of "electric shock" can induce ventricular fibrillation if applied directly to excitable areas of the heart. The most stringent current restrictions (10 microamperes) apply to conditions in which there are direct electrically conductive paths present from the exterior to the body to the heart, such as an intracardiac catheter. For normal applications using external electrodes, currents as high as 5 milliamperes can be tolerated without risk. However, in the design of a piece of equipment, it is best to yield to the most rigorous application.

Since a voltage difference is a prerequisite for an electrical current to flow, one only has to ensure that the patient and everything in contact with him are at the same voltage. The obvious way to achieve this is to have everything grounded. If this is applied correctly, there is no doubt that patient safety is assured. However, it is often far from easy to ground everything. Many electrical outlets are of the older, two-slot variety and *do not* have a grounding connection. The latter-type outlet should be avoided or at the very least adapted for a grounding connection via the receptacle plate. However, even if the outlet is of the three-prolonged grounded variety, what assurance is there that the ground conductor in the building wiring is not broken at some point? Also, if the wiring is correct, there may be enough equipment connected to the supply relying on the same ground conductor so that current flowing in the ground wire makes its voltage no longer truly "zero." It is not uncommon in tall buildings to find two "grounds" on different circuits 1/2 volt different from each other, even in the same room. Two pieces of equipment, one on each circuit, would then cause 500 microamperes of current to flow through a patient (assuming a minimal body resistance of 1000 ohms) if he were connected to both.

Even properly grounded plugs provide incomplete patient safety; therefore, the clinician must rely on the manufacturer providing safeguards in the apparatus itself. For example, most of the potential hazard arises from a damaged power transformer since there is always capacitive current flowing between the windings. Proper shielding of the power transformer (which would be noted in the manufacturing specifications) will eliminate this danger. More complete patient safety is provided in some species of apparatus by having the input terminals connected internally to an isolation transformer, which effectively isolates the patient from such potential hazard points as the power line, ground, and instrument chassis.

If your instrumentation does not provide adequate patient safeguards, you should consider fusing the input terminals. This simply involves placing 5 or 10 milliamp *extra fast blow* fuses in series with the contact lens electrode and reference electrode leads. A convenient way of doing this is to have the fuses inside the terminal function box. In using fuses, remember that it loads the amplifier (depending on the value fuses used) up to 1000 ohms higher than unfused inputs. Be sure, there-

111

fore, that the input resistance of the scope of polygraph is great enough to accommodate the increased load. Input resistances of 1 to 10 megohms are typically provided in modern amplifiers and easily handle the small additional load imposed by the fuse. Be aware, however, that additional resistance may decrease the high frequency response of the amplifier. While such losses should not impair the fidelity of any of the ERG components, this point should be checked by comparing amplifier response to generated wave-forms of 100 to 300 Hz with and without the fuses in the circuit.

Appendix D
Color Vision Testing

The application of physiological processes associated with color vision has only recently been appreciated in the clinical field. The definitive finding of three separate types of cone receptors and the recent application of receptive fields and their role in color vision have served to amalgamate the Helmholtz and Hering schools.

1. PHYSIOLOGY OF COLOR VISION

The perception of color is a cortical response to specific physical stimuli received by the eyes. A narrow band of the electromagnetic spectrum, wavelengths between 400 and 700 nm, are capable of passing through the transparent portions of the eye and being absorbed by visual pigments contained in the outer segments of cone receptors. Any cone contains one of three types of photolabile pigment, each absorbing a particular range of wavelengths centered in the short, middle, or long wavelength region. Thus, we designate blue-, green-, and red-sensitive cones as the basic initiators of color vision.

Selective wavelength absorption by cones provides only the crude beginning of an elaborate neurophysiological mechanism for color vision. The visual cortex, with which retinal cones must ultimately communicate, recognizes only trains of all-or-none action potentials. What is the mechanism by which specific wavelengths are transformed into an unambiguous telegraphic message recognizable as a "color?" A direct solution envisioned by the 19th century scientist, Thomas Young, simply assigned specific optic nerve fibers to sympathetically resonate to specific wavelengths. This appealing theory could not be sustained when it was shown that changing only the intensity of the light stimulus greatly changes the optic nerve firing pattern. Clearly, a mechanism that cannot distinguish between intensity and wavelength is inappropriate for reliable color discrimination. A plausible neurophysiological model for color perception was, in fact, only recently formulated and is based on the fact that each major portion of the visual pathway, retina, midbrain, and cortex is organized into functional units called "receptive fields." A receptive field is a group of neural elements designed to detect differences in stimulus configuration. Thus, there are receptive fields organized to detect differences in brightness, patterns, motion, and color. The fields usually consist of excitatory and inhibitory regions set up so that one region concentrically surrounds the other; a ganglion cell of the retina will increase its firing rate if the central (excitatory) portion of the photoreceptor field is stimulated and decreases its firing if the surround (inhibitory) portion of the field is stimulated. Such a receptive field would be classed as an on-center off-surround type. Receptive fields for color are similarly organized, except that the excitatory and inhibitory portions of the field are wavelength dependent, producing what is in effect an opponent-color unit. Thus a red on-center, green off-surround cortical cell would increase its firing rate if reddish light fell near the field center on the retina and would decrease its firing rate if greenish light fell on the surrounding areas of the field. The final requirement of a color detection mechanism is satisfied in that even slight changes in wavelength are translated into a detectable increase or decrease in firing rate.

Each cone pigment absorbs a broad

113

range of wavelengths, although each is not absorbed equally. A red-sensitive pigment, for example, would absorb greater amounts of red and lesser amounts from the other spectral regions. If this red-sensitive cone were directly connected to a ganglion cell and stimulated with a whole range of wavelengths, it would be possible to produce the same spike firing rate by simply adjusting the intensity of any wavelength. Clearly, to have a ganglion cell discriminate between wavelength and intensity requires another factor: the presence of at least one other type of cone pigment, for instance, a green-sensitive one, the output of which feeds into the same ganglion cell. Under these circumstances, the ganglion cell receives a signal derived from the two cones, and no amount of intensity manipulation can now "match wave lengths" since each pigment is absorbing quite different numbers of quanta based on their intrinsic sensitivities. Thus, a minimal requirement for color discrimination is the presence of at least two kinds of cone photopigment. In the following part it will be learned that for normal color vision, all three, red-, green-, and blue-sensitive cones, must be functioning.

Obviously, if one is only concerned with foveal receptive fields, the rod contribution to the color field can be neglected. However, ganglion cells just outside the fovea do receive rod input, and this rod input must necessarily increase the farther from the fovea the stimulus is located. Since rods contain the visual pigment rhodopsin (which itself absorbs a broad range of wavelengths centered around the blue-green region of the spectrum), do rods also provide additional color information when activated with cones? It has been shown that if a ganglion cell of the retina that has both cone and rod input is tested in the dark-adapted state and in the presence of a light background, cones preempt neural activity under the light (photopic) condition and the rods dominate the receptive field output under dark (scotopic) conditions.[126] This experiment is another demonstration of the Purkinje shift and, in addition, emphasizes the fact that rods do not appear to contribute to the mediation of color perception.

2. CLASSIFICATION AND TESTING OF COLOR VISION ANOMALIES

It should be clearly understood that specific aspects of the physical stimuli we call "visible light" have behavioral responses associated with them. The response characteristics of the stimuli are the accepted verbal labels that are generally agreed on by a vast majority of normals. Stimuli and response variables can be related as shown in Table D.1.

Table D.2 shows one means of classifying color vision defects. It is based on a laboratory testing method called color matching. Briefly, a subject is asked to match an unknown wavelength by manipulating a mixture of three (known) standard wavelengths. A normal observer requires all three (red, green, and blue) standards to make the match and, hence, is classified as trichromatic. A small percentage of color abnormals require only two of the three standards to perform a match with an unknown color and are called dichromats. From the data of such studies it was inferred, and later proved, that three types of dichromats exist: those lacking the red-sensitive, green-sensitive, or blue-sensitive photopigment in their cones.

Persons with a red-green deficiency related to the red-sensitive pigment loss were historically described first, and the conditions were simply referred to as protanopia, literally "an absence of vision of the first sort." There is a second type of red-green dichromacy involving a green-sensitive pigment loss, and it is known as deuteranopia, "absence of vision of the second kind." Blue-yellow color blindness, the third form, completes the dichromacy class and is referred to as "tritanopia." Although protanopes and deuteranopes both represent forms of red-green deficiency, they can be clearly distinguished from each other as indicated in Table D.2. One needs only to remember that it is the protanope that has a luminosity loss in the

Table D.1
The Stimulus and Response Correlates of Color

Stimulus	Response
Wavelength	Hue or color
Radiant flux (quanta per unit time from a unit area of radiating emitter)	Intensity, brightness, luminance
Saturation	Depth of color (e.g., dark blue vs. light blue)

Table D.2
Color Vision Deficits Classified by Color Matching

I. Trichromat: requires all 3 primaries for matching an unknown color
II. Anomalous trichromat: uses anomalous amounts of primaries for color matches
    Protanomalous uses more red than normal
    Deuteranomalous uses more green than normal
    Tritanomalous uses more blue than normal
        Note: Both protan and deutan are red-green weak. Difference is that protan shows slight luminosity loss in red end of spectrum, while deutan maintains luminosity with range of R-G confusion.
    Genetic lesion, probably substitution of anomalous protein portion of photopigment molecule
III. Dichromat: requires only 2 of 3 primaries for color match
    Protanope: loss of red-sensitive pigment
    Deuteranope: loss of green-sensitive pigment
    Tritanope: loss of blue-sensitive pigment
    Genetic lesion: In protan, presumptive "red" cone manufactures green- (or blue-) sensitive pigment. Similar substitutions for deutan and tritan
        Note: There is no acuity loss in above because all cones are filled with 2 of 3 possible pigments.
IV. Monochromat: requires only 1 of the 3 primaries to match any unknown
    Rod monochromat (typical achromatopsia): congenital, stationary, generalized cone loss, including fovea
    Syndrome: low visual acuity, absent color vision, photophobia, nystagmus, *absent flicker ERG*
    Cone monochromat (atypical achromat): has only 1 type of cone, e.g., "green-cone monochromat" or "blue-cone monochromat." Since at least 2 kinds of cones are required to discriminate colors, the patient is functionally as much an achromat as "coneless" form.
    Syndrome: no color sense, normal acuity, no nystagmus or photophobia, and *normal flicker ERG.*

end of the spectrum while the deuteranope (presumably because of the flanking position of the remaining blue- and red-sensitive pigment to the missing green-sensitive pigment) shows little luminosity change across the spectrum. A deuteranope could easily confuse the color of cherries with the leaves whereas the protanope would always see the cherries as much darker than the green leaves.

The class of anomalous trichromats makes up the largest group of color-deficient persons. These individuals require three primaries to match an unknown but use them in "anomalous" amounts, compared to normal trichromats. They are usually said to be "color weak" rather than "color blind." Each of the anomalous trichromats has an analogous defect to the dichromats. Thus, the protanomalous patient is "red-weak," requiring more red in a red-green mixture to match a yellow.

While the dichromat represents an actual lack of one kind of cone pigment, the anomalous trichromat has not been shown to have a "diluted" amount of red-, green-, or blue-sensitive pigment; rather, the genetic lesion in these color anomalies appears to be a subtle alteration in the protein (opsin) portion of the visual pigment molecule. The slight shift in the maxima of the absorption curves of the affected pigment is held responsible for the subtle color perception defect.

There are two forms of "achromatopsia," and although both leave the affected individual completely without color discrimination (technically "monochromats," since any spectral color can be matched to any one of the three standards solely by intensity adjustments), they are two quite separate entities.

The rod monochromat is born without functioning cones in the retina, and such a loss accounts for the associated symptoms of low visual acuity, absent color vision, aversion to bright lights, and nystagmus. The generalized loss of cones in this condition is unequivocally shown by the absent ERG response to rapid (>20/sec) flicker stimuli.

Cone monochromatism represents an achromatopsia with no other symptoms. Persons affected with this extremely rare condition have no hue discrimination but normal acuity and no photophobia or nystagmus. Cone monochromats do indeed have cones, but all the cones contain the same visual pigment. Exactly why a person with only one cone pigment is achromatic has already been discussed, but there is a simple demonstration to emphasize the point. Hold a narrow band of colored filter (preferably in interference type) in front of one eye. Depending on the dominant wavelength of the filter, the world will look blue, green, etc. The point is that although everything is suffused

Table D.3
Color Vision Tests

Test	Mode of operation	Defects detected	Sensitivity/quantification	Ease of administration
Ishihara	Color confusion	R-G only	Extremely sensitive/nil	Difficult for preschool children and low IQ
AO H-R-R	Saturation	R-G, B-Y	Will miss very mild R-G defects/good classification	Excellent for all ages
Farnsworth Panel D-15	Color confusion	R-G, B-Y	Will only detect severe anomalous trichromatopsia and dichromatopsia/good classification	Easy to administer
Farnsworth-Munsell 100 hue	Hue discrimination	R-G, B-Y, and normal "color insensitive"	Extremely sensitive/classify by error scoring	Tedious to administer
Nagel anomaloscope	Luminosity match	R-G only	Very sensitive/classify by anomaly (R-G) quotient	Requires patient cooperation
Sloan achromatopsia test	Hue-brightness match	Achromatopsia only	Grossly sensitive/very incomplete achromatopsia pass	Easy to administer

Note: All tests, with exception of Nagel anomaloscope, are to be administered under an Illuminant C source such as provided by a Macbeth Easel Lamp.

with a "color," it is not possible to correctly name the color of any object. Only previous, color-normal experience allows the correct label of the transmitted filter wavelength. This is denied the cone monochromat, and he is totally without the means to discriminate hue. The one congenital color defect having symptoms of poor acuity and achromatopsia, (rod monochromatism) must always be considered in making the differential diagnosis in such patients, although the history of poor vision from birth and the associated nystagmus usually suffice to make the distinction.

3. TESTING FOR COLOR VISION DEFECTS

a. All dichromats and anomalous trichromats see a desaturated spectrum. The dichromats, in particular, see all colors as "washed out," compared to normal.

b. Dichromats and anomalous trichromats have poor hue discrimination; thus, such color defectives require a greater than normal change in wavelength in order to sense a hue change.

c. All color abnormals confuse pairs of colors in the visible spectrum. Exactly which pairs are color confused may be diagnostic for a particular defect, and this phenomenon is used as the basis for several of the tests listed in Table D.3.

d. Luminosity losses in the spectrum are subtle for the anomalous trichromats, obvious for two kinds of dichromat (protan and tritan), and pronounced for the monochromat. An instrument called a Nagel anomaloscope designed for office use, allows the patient to match spectral yellow to a red-green mixture by varying the brightness of the yellow test field. It is a sensitive indicator for both dichromacy and anomalous trichromacy of the protan and deutan types.

Table D.3 shows how each kind of color test uses one of the above four facts as a basis for classifying the various color vision anomalies. For office use, either the AOH-R-R or Ishihara plates are employed for screening purposes. If a defect is found but is not clearly classifiable, another test such as the Farnsworth Panel D-15 should be used to obtain further diagnostic information.

Distinguishing acquired disorders of color vision can be confusing. It is many years since the Köllner law was enunciated, i.e., inner retinal layer diseases produce blue-yellow defects. Further research on this phenomenon shows it to be just as often an inaccurate indicator for diagnosis, as it occasionally proves itself correct. What is unmistakable, however, is that acquired color blinds are almost consistently unclassifiable as to defect type on any particular test. This fact, taken together with the observation that acquired color defects are also associated with visual acuity loss, should alert the examiner.

Appendix E

Dark Adaptometry and Retinal Profiles

Measuring the course of dark adaptation after exposure to a bright light affords the clinician an opportunity to evaluate several vital retinal functions. These include quantitative estimates of cone and rod participation in the visual process, their absolute sensitivities, and the recovery time for the two systems after light desensitization. Commercial instruments are available for such testing, but the general principles outlined below apply to any apparatus constructed for the purpose.

After exposure to an intense preadapting light (5–7 minutes using a diffuse 3000 millilambert source with dilated pupil is sufficient), the room lights are extinguished, and the patient's gaze is directed toward an illuminated fixation point while a 1 or 2° diameter stimulus is placed in a retinal area located about 15° temporal to the fovea. Every minute or so the examiner records the intensity of the stimulus light, which just produces a threshold response from the patient. The *solid line* (Fig. E.1) represents a curve drawn through the determined threshold values and forms the typical two-branched curve of dark adaptation. The first branch represents the fast adaptation of the cone system. It reaches a plateau in about 5 minutes and maintains a steady threshold value for another few minutes after which the rod system intervenes (rod-cone break) and forms the more slowly adapting rod branch. The latter takes about 20 minutes in the dark to reach its steady threshold level. The two plateaus are the absolute thresholds of the cone and rod systems, and the time each branch takes to reach the plateau is a measure of its rate of adaptation.

If the stimulus were placed inside the foveal region, little of the second (rod) branch would appear. If the retina had a defective scotopic system, such as occurs in typical congenital nyctalopia, a single (cone) branch would be produced, even 15° from the fovea[96] (*upper dashed curve* in Fig. E.1). Conversely, if the patient were a rod monochromat, there would be no cone contribution to the curve, and a single-branched curve representing solely rod function would be obtained.[33] It should be emphasized that the cone and rod sensitivity in only *one specific area* of the retina

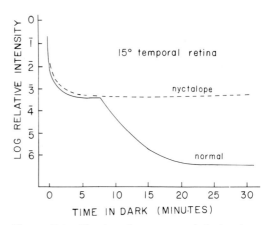

Figure E.1 Plotting the course of dark adaptation. After exposing the eye to a bright light (about 3000 mililamberts) for several minutes, the patient is directed to fixate a small red light located so that the stimulus falls 15° temporal to the fovea. The stimulus intensity required which just elicits a threshold response is determined each minute and plotted on the *abscissa* time scale. The normal eye produces a bipartite function, with the cone-rod "break" occurring at about 7 min. Patients deficient in rod function, such as the congenital nyctalope, will lack the lower (rod) portion of the curve.

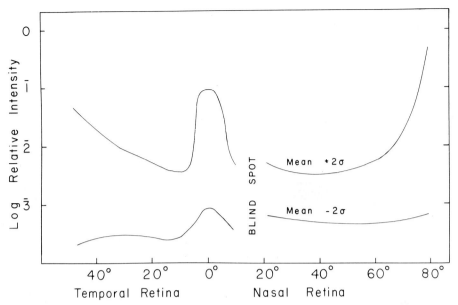

Figure E.2 A profile of retinal sensitivity is obtained by measuring intensity thresholds across the dark-adapted retina. The shape of the profile indicates that the fovea is less sensitive than more peripheral portions of the retina. Most normals fall within the ±2 SD threshold boundaries indicated.

has been measured with this technique—in the present instance, a small area 15° from the fovea. To determine thresholds across the retina or in any meridian (retinal profiles), it is only necessary to dark-adapt a patient fully and measure thresh-old values at specific distances (say in 5° steps from the fovea). Commercial dark adaptometers such as the Goldmann-Weekers model have such a provision. Figure E.2 shows a retinal profile obtained in the horizontal meridian.

References

GENERAL

Arden, G. B. *The Retina-Neurophysiology in the eye*, edited by H. Davson, Vol. 2A, Chap. 7. Academic Press, New York, 1976.

Armington, J. C. *The Electroretinogram*. Academic Press, New York, 1974.

Berson, E. L. Electrical phenomena in the retina. In: *Adler's Physiology of the Eye*, edited by R. Moses, p. 466. St. Louis, C. V. Mosby, 1981.

Electrophysiology and psychophysics: Their use in ophthalmic diagnosis. Int. Ophthalmol. Clin., *20*, 1980.

1. Riggs, L. A.: Continuous and reproducible records of the human retina. Proc. Soc. Exp. Biol. 48:204, 1941.
2. Østerberg, G.: Topography of the layer of rods and cones in the human retina. Acta Ophthalmol. 13 (Suppl. 6), 1935.
3. Fry, G. A., and Bartley, S. H.: The relation of stray light in the eye to the retinal action potential. Am. J. Physiol. 111:335, 1935.
4. Brown, K. T., Watanabe, K., and Murakami, M.: The early and late receptor potentials of monkey cones and rods. Cold Spring Harbor Symp. Quant. Biol. 30:457, 1965.
5. Gouras, P., and Carr, R. E.: Light-induced DC responses of monkey retina before and after central retinal artery interruption. Invest. Ophthalmol. 4:310, 1965.
6. Karpe, G.: The basis of clinical electroretinography. Acta Ophthalmol. 4 (Suppl. 24), 1945.
7. Hagins, W. A., Penn, R. D., and Yoshikami, S.: Dark current and photocurrent in retinal rods. Biophys. J. 10:380, 1970.
8. Murakami, M., and Kaneko, A. Subcomponents of PIII in cold-blooded vertebrate retinas. Nature 210:103, 1966.
9. Ripps, H., Shakib, M., and MacDonald, E. D.: Peroxidase uptake by photoreceptor terminals of the skate retina. J. Cell Biol. 70:86, 1976.
10. Werblin, F. S., and Dowling, J. E.: Organization of the retina of the mudpuppy Necturus maculosus. II. Intracellular recording. J. Neurophysiol. 32:339, 1969.
11. Miller, R. F., and Dowling, J. E.: Intracellular responses of the Müller (glial) cells of mudpuppy retina: Their relation to b-wave of the electroretinogram. J. Neurophysiol. 33:323–341, 1970.
12. Kline, R. P., Ripps, H., and Dowling, J. E.: Generation of b-wave currents in the skate retina. Proc. Natl. Acad. Sci. USA, 75:5727, 1978.
13. Szamier, R. B., Ripps, H., and Chappell, R. Changes in ERG b-wave and Müller cell structure induced by x-aminoadipic acid. Neurosci. Lett. 21:307, 1981.
14. Gouras, P.: Electroretinography: Some basic principles. Invest. Ophthalmol. 9:557, 1970.
15. Siegel, I. M. A ganzfeld content lens electrode. Am. J. Ophthalmol. 80:296, 1975.
16. Armington, J. C., Tepas, D. I., Kropfl, W. J., and Hengst, W. H.: Summation of retinal potentials. J. Opt. Soc. Am. 51:877, 1961.
17. Aiba, T. S., Alpern, M., and Maaseidvaag, F.: The electroretinogram evoked by the excitation of human foveal cones. J. Physiol. 189:43, 1967.
18. Riggs, L. A., Johnson, E. P., Schick, A. M. L.: Electrical responses of the human eye to moving stimulus patterns. Science 144:567, 1964.
19. Armington, J. C.: The electroretinogram, the visual evoked potential and the area-luminance relation. Vision Res. 8:263, 1968.
20. Arden, G. B.: A gold foil electrode: extending the horizons for clinical electroretinography. Invest. Ophthalmol. 18:421, 1979.
21. Cummings, R. W., and Kaluzne, S. J.: An improved electrode for electroretinography: Design and standardization. Am. J. Optom. Physiol. Opt. 55:719, 1978.
22. Sokol, S., and Nadler, D.: Simultaneous electroretinograms and visually evoked potentials from adult amblyopes in response to a pattern stimulus. Invest. Ophthalmol. Visual. Sci. 18:848, 1979.
23. Arden, G. B., Vaegan, Hogg, C. R., Powell, D. J., and Carter R. M.: Pattern ERGs are abnormal in many amblyopes. Trans. Ophthalmol. Soc. U.K. 100, in press, 1979.

24. Hess, R. F.: Contrast sensitivity assessment of functional amblyopia in humans. Trans. Ophthalmol. Soc. U.K. 99:319, 1979.

25. Sokol, S. An electrodiagnostic index of macular degeneration. Use of a checkerboard pattern stimulus. Arch. Opthalmol. 88:619, 1972.

26. Arden, G. B., Barrada, A., and Kelsey, J. H.: New clinical test of retinal function based upon the standing potential of the eye. Br. J. Ophthalmol. 46:449, 1962.

27. Adams, A.: The normal electro-oculogram (EOG). Acta Ophthalmol. (Separatum) 51:551, 1973.

28. Arden, G. B., and Kelsey, J. H.: Changes produced by light in the standing potential of the human eye. J. Physiol. 161:189, 1962.

29. Fishman, G. A., et al.: Electro-oculogram testing in fundus flavimaculatus. Arch. Ophthalmol. 97:1896, 1979.

30. Oakley, B.: Potassium and the photoreceptor-dependent pigment epithelial hyperpolarization. J. Gen. Physiol. 70:405, 1977.

31. Steinberg, R., and Niemeyer, G.: Light peak of cat DC electroretinogram not generated by a change in $(K^+)_o$. Invest. Ophthalmol. Visual Sci. 20:414, 1981.

32. Nilsson, S. E. G., and Skoog, K.: Covariation of the simultaneously recorded c-wave and standing potential of the human eye. Acta Ophthalmol. 53:721, 1975.

33. Carr, R. E., and Siegel, I. M.: Electrophysiologic aspects of several retinal diseases. Am. J. Ophthalmol. 58:95, 1964.

34. Sokol, S.: Visually evoked potentials: Theory, techniques and clinical applications. Surv. Ophthalmol. 21:18, 1976.

35. Arden, G. B., Faulkner, D. J., and Mair, C.: A versatile television pattern generator for visual evoked potentials. In: Visual Evoked Potentials in Man, edited by J. E. Desmedt. Oxford, Clarendon Press, 1977.

36. Sjöstrand, J., and Frisen, L.: Contrast sensitivity in macular disease. Acta Ophthalmol. 55:509, 1977.

37. Hess, R., and Woo, G.: Vision through cataracts. Invest. Ophthalmol. Visual Sci. 17:428, 1978.

38. Arden, G. B.: The visual evoked response in ophthalmology. Proc. R. Soc. Med. 66:1037, 1973.

39. Fishman, G. A., Fishman, M., and Maggiano, J.: Macular lesions associated with retinitis pigmentosa. Arch. Ophthalmol. 95:798, 1977.

40. Fetkenhour, C. L., et al.: Cystoid macular edema in retinitis pigmentosa. Trans. Am. Acad. Ophthalmol. Otolaryngol. 83:515, 1977.

41. Geltzer, A. I., and Berson, E. L.: Fluorescein angiography of hereditary retinal degenerations. Arch. Ophthalmol. 81:766, 1969.

42. Vernon, M.: Usher's syndrome—Deafness and progressive blindness. J. Chron. Dis. 22:133, 1969.

43. Goode, R. L., Rafaty, F. M., and Simmons, F. B.: Hearing loss in retinitis pigmentosa. Pediatrics 40:875, 1967.

44. Bateman, J. B., et al.: Heterogeneity of retinal degeneration and hearing impairment syndromes. Am. J. Ophthalmol. 90:755, 1980.

45. Krill, A. E. Hereditary Retinal and Choroidal Diseases, Vol. II, pp. 481–482. Harper & Row, Hagerstown, Md., 1977.

46. Jay, B.: Hereditary aspects of pigmentary retinopathy. Trans. Ophthalmol. Soc. U.K. 92:193, 1972.

47. Berson, E. L., Rosen, J. B., and Simonoff, E. A.: ERG testing as an aid in detection of carriers of X-chromosome-linked retinitis pigmentosa. Am. J. Ophthalmol. 87:460, 1979.

48. Berson, E. L., Gouras, P., and Hoff, M.: Temporal aspects of the electroretinogram. Arch. Ophthalmol. 81:207, 1969.

49. Lauber, H.: Die sogenannte Retinitis punctata albescens. Klin. Monatsbl. Augenheilkd. 48:133, 1910.

50. Francois, J.: Heredity in Ophthalmology, edited by C.V. Mosby, p. 457. St. Louis, 1961.

51. Leber, T.: Über Retinitis pigmentosa und angeborene Amaurose. Graefe. Arch. Opthalmol. 15:1, 1869.

52. Mizuno, K., et al.: Leber's congenital amaurosis. Am. J. Ophthalmol. 83:32, 1977.

53. Margolis, S., Scher, B. M., and Carr, R. E.: Macular colobomas in Leber's congenital amaurosis. Am. J. Ophthalmol. 83:27, 1977.

54. Schappert-Kimmijser, J., Henkes, H. E., and van den Borsch, J.: Amaurosis congenita (Leber). Arch. Opthalmol. 61:211, 1959.

55. Sorsby, A., and Williams, C. E.: Retinal aplasia as a clinical entity. Br. Med. J. 2:293, 1960.

56. Alström, C. H., and Olson, O.: Heredo-retinopathio congenitalis monohybrida recessive autosomalis. Hereditas 43:1, 1957.

57. Franceschetti, A., Francois, J., and Babel, J.: Chorioretinal Heredo-degenerations, p. 316. Charles C Thomas, Springfield, Ill., 1974.

58. Bjork, A., Lindblom, U., and Wadensten, L.: Retinal degeneration in hereditary ataxia. J. Neurol. Neurosurg. Psychiatry 19:186, 1956.

59. Kurstjens, I. H.: Choroideremia and gyrate atrophy of the choroid and retina. Doc. Ophthalmol. 19:1, 1965.

60. Noble, K. G., Carr, R. E., and Siegel, I. M.: Fluorescein angiography of the hereditary choroidal dystrophies. Br. J. Ophthalmol. 61:43, 1977.

61. Lyon, M. F.: Sex chromatin and gene action in mammalian X-chromosome. Am. J. Hum. Genet. 14:135, 1962.

62. Simell, O., and Takki, K.: Raised plasma-ornithine and gyrate atrophy of the choroid and retina. Lancet 1:1031, 1973.

63. Valle, D., Kaiser-Kupfer, M. I., and Del Valle, L.

A.: Gyrate atrophy of the choroid and retina. Deficiency of ornithine amino transferase in transformed lymphocytes. Proc. Natl. Acad. Sci. USA 74:5159, 1977.

64. McCulloch, C., and Marliss, D.: Gyrate atrophy of the choroid and retina: Clinical, ophthalmologic, and biochemical considerations. Tr. Am. Ophthalmol. Soc. 73:153, 1975.

65. Weleber, R. A., Kennaway, N. G., and Brust, N. R. R.: Vitamin B6 in management of gyrate atrophy of choroid and retina. Lancet 2:1213, 1978.

66. Kaiser-Kupfer, M. I., DeMonasterio, F. M., et al.: Gyrate atrophy of the choroid and retina: Improved visual function following reduction of plasma ornithine by diet. Science 210:1128, 1980.

67. Welch, R. B.: Bietti's tapetoretinal degeneration with marginal corneal dystrophy: Crystalline retinopathy. Trans. Am. Ophthalmol. Soc. 75: 164, 1977.

68. Carr, R. E., and Siegel, I. M.: The vitreo-tapetoretinal degenerations. Arch. Ophthalmol. 84:436, 1970.

69. Stickler, G. B., et al.: Hereditary progressive arthro-ophthalmopathy. Proc. Mayo Clin. 40: 433, 1965.

70. Blair, N. P., et al.: Hereditary progressive arthro-ophthalmopathy of Stickler. Am. J. Ophthalmol. 88:876, 1979.

71. Potts, A. M.: Uveal pigment and phenothiazine compounds. Trans. Am. Ophthalmol. Soc. 60: 517, 1962.

72. Burian, H. M., and Fletcher, M. C.: Visual functions in patients with retinal pigmentary degeneration following use of N.P. 207. Arch. Ophthalmol. 60:612, 1958.

73. Henkind, P., and Rothfield, N.: Ocular abnormalities in patients treated with antimalarial drugs. N. Engl. J. Med. 269:433, 1963.

74. Carr, R. E., et al.: Ocular toxicity of antimalarial drugs: Long-term follow-up. Am. J. Ophthalmol. 66:738, 1968.

75. Arden, G. B., Friedmann, A., and Kolb, H.: Anticipation of chloroquine retinopathy. Lancet 1: 1164, 1962.

76. Carr, R. E., and Siegel, I. M.: Unilateral retinitis pigmentosa. Arch. Ophthalmol. 90:21, 1973.

77. Knave, B.: Electroretinography in eyes with retained intraocular metallic foreign bodies. Acta Ophthalmol. (Suppl. 100), 1969.

78. Declercq, S. S., Meredith, P. C. A., and Rosenthal, A. R.: Experimental siderosis in the rabbit: correlation between electroretinography and histopathology. Arch. Ophthalmol. 95:1051, 1977.

79. Gass, J. D. M., et al.: Diffuse unilateral subacute neuroretinitis. Ophthalmology 85:520, 1978.

80. Pearlman, J. T., Heckenlively, J. R., and Bastek, J. V.: Progressive nature of pigmented paraven-

ous retinochoroidal atrophy. Am. J. Ophthalmol. 85:215, 1978.

81. Klien, B. A., and Krill, A. E.: Fundus flavimaculatus: clinical, functional, and histopathologic observations. Am. J. Ophthalmol. 64:3, 1967.

82. Eagle, R. C., Lucier, A. C., Bernardino, V. B., and Yanoff, M.: Retinal pigment epithelial abnormalities in fundus flavimaculatus; A light and electron microscopic study. Ophthalmology 87: 1189, 1981.

83. Bassem, F. A., and Kornzweig, A. L.: Malformation of the erythrocytes in a case of atypical retinitis pigmentosa. Blood 5:318, 1950.

84. Salt, H. B., Wolff, O. H., Lloyd, J. K., Fosbrooke, A. S., Cameron, A. H., and Hubble, D. V.: On having no betalipoprotein: a syndrome comprising a-betalipoproteinemia, acanthocytosis, and steatorrhoea. Lancet 2:325, 1960.

85. Ways, P., Reed, C. F., and Hanahan, D. J.: Red-cell and plasma lipids in acanthocytosis. J. Clin. Invest. 42:1248, 1963.

86. Gouras, P., Carr, R. E., and Gunkel, R. D.: Retinitis pigmentosa in abetalipoproteinemia: Effects of vitamin A. Invest. Ophthalmol., 10:784, 1971.

87. Refsum, S.: Heredopathia atactica polyneuritiformis: A familial syndrome not hitherto described. Acta Psychiatr. Scand. 38:1, 1946.

88. Richterich, R., Kählke, W., von Mechelen, P., and Rossi, E.: Refsum's Syndrome: Ein angeborener Defekt im Lipid-Stoffwechsel mit Speicherung von 3,7,11,15-Tetramethyl-Hexadecansaure. Klin. Wochenschr., 41:800, 1963.

89. Baum, J., Tannenbaum, M., and Kolodny, E.: Refsum's syndrome with corneal involvement. Am. J. Ophthalmol. 60:699, 1965.

90. Masters-Thomas, A., et al.: Heredopathia atactica polyneuritiformis (Refsum's disease). I. Clinical features and dietary management. J. Hum. Nutr. 34:245, 1980.

91. Hooft, C., et al.: Familial hypolipidaemia and retarded development without steatorrhoea: Another inborn error of metabolism? Helv. Paediatr. Acta 17:1, 1962.

92. Copenhaver, R., and Goodman, G.: The ERG in infantile, late infantile, and juvenile amaurotic family idiocy. Arch. Ophthalmol. 63:559, 1960.

93. Sidman, R. L.: Histochemical studies in photoreceptor cells. Ann. N.Y. Acad. Sci. 72:162, 1958.

94. Franceschetti, A., and Klein, D.: Les manifestations tapéto-rétiniennes et leur importance clinique et génétique dans les hérédo-ataxies. Rev. Oto-Neuro-Ophthalmol. (Paris) 20:109, 1948.

95. Kearns, T. P.: External ophthalmoplegic, pigmentary degeneration of the retina, and cardiomyopathy. Trans. Am. Ophthalmol. Soc. 63:559, 1965.

96. Carr, R. E., et al.: Rhodopsin and the electrical

activity of the retina in congenital nightblindness. Invest. Ophthalmol. 5:497, 1966.

97. Carr, R. E., and Gouras, P.: Oguchi's disease. Arch. Ophthalmol. 73:646, 1965.

98. Carr, R. E.: Congenital stationary nightblindness. Trans. Am. Ophthalmol. Soc. 72:448, 1974.

99. Carr, R. E., and Ripps, H.: Rhodopsin kinetics and rod adaptation in Oguchi's disease. Invest. Ophthalmol. 6:426, 1967.

100. Carr, R. E., Ripps, H., and Siegel, I. M.: Visual pigment kinetics and adaptation in fundus albipunctatus. In: *Documenta Ophthalmologica Proceedings Series XIth ISCERG Symposium*, p. 193. 1974.

101. Blackwell, H. R., and Blackwell, O. M.: Rod and cone receptor mechanisms in typical and atypical congenital achromatopsia. Vis. Res. 1:62, 1961.

102. Weale, R. A.: Some aspects of total colour-blindness. Trans. Ophthalmol. Soc. U.K. 73:241, 1953.

103. Siegel, I. M., and Smith, B. F.: Acquired cone dysfunction. Arch. Ophthalmol. 77:8, 1967.

104. Siegel, I. M., and Arden, G. B.: The effects of drugs on color vision. In: *Drugs and Sensory Functions*, edited by A. Herxheimer, pp. 210–228. London, J. A. Churchill, 1968.

105. Carr, R. E., and Siegel, I. M.: Ocular disorders associated with albinism. In: *The Retinal Pigment Epithelium*, edited by K. Zinn and M. F. Marmour, pp. 413–423. Cambridge, Mass., Harvard University Press, 1979.

106. Siegel, I. M.: Ophthalmological findings in tyrosinase positive oculocutaneous albinism. Perspect. Ophthalmol. 3:17, 1979.

107. Goodman, A., Ripps, H., and Siegel, I. M.: Sex-linked ocular disorders. Arch. Ophthalmol. 73:387, 1965.

108. Henkind, P., Carr, R. E., and Siegel, I. M.: Early chloroquine retinopathy: clinical and functional findings. Arch. Ophthalmol. 71:157, 1964.

109. Deutman, A. F.: Electro-oculography in families with vitelliform dystrophy of the fovea. Arch. Ophthalmol. 81:305, 1969.

110. Deutman, A. F., et al.: Butterfly-shaped pigment dystrophy of the fovea. Arch. Ophthalmol. 83:558, 1970.

111. Maffei, L., and Fiorentino, A.: Electroretinographic responses to alternating gratings before and after section of the optic nerve. Science 211:953, 1981.

112. Nelson, R., Zrenner, E., and Gouras, P.: Patterned stimuli reveal spatial organization in the electroretinogram. Proceedings of the XVI of ISCEV, Symposium, pp. 161–169. Japanese Journal of Ophthalmology, Tokyo, 1979.

113. Bodis-Wollner, I., et al.: Visual association cortex and vision in man: Pattern-evoked occipital potentials in a blind boy. Science 198:629, 1977.

114. Wachtmeister, L.: On the oscillatory potentials of the human ERG in light and dark adaptation. IV. Effect of adaptation to short flashes of light. Time interval and intensity of conditioning flashes. A Fourier analysis. Acta Ophthalmol. 50:250, 1972.

115. Yonemura, D., Tsuzuki, K., and Aoki, T.: The clinical importance of oscillatory potentials in the human ERG. Acta Ophthalmol. (Suppl. 70): 115, 1962.

116. Gjötterberg, M. The ERG in diabetic retinopathy. A clinical study and a critical survey. Acta Ophthalmol. 52:521, 1974.

117. Yonemura, D.: Study of the human ERG. New approaches to ophthalmic electrodiagnosis. Proceedings of the XVI Symposium of ISCEV, edited by Y. Tazawa, pp. 1–13. Japanese Journal of Ophthalmology, Tokyo, 1979.

118. Ogden, T. E.: The oscillatory waves of the primate electroretinogram. Vision Res. 13:1059, 1973.

119. Wachtmeister, L., and Dowling, J. E.: The oscillatory potentials of the mudpuppy retina. Invest. Ophthalmol. 17:1176, 1978.

120. Fuller, D. G., Knighton, R. W., and Machemer, R.: Bright-flash ERG for the evaluation of eyes with opaque vitreous. Am. J. Ophthalmol. 80:214, 1975.

121. Mandelbaum, S., et al.: Bright-flash electroretinography and vitreous hemorrhage. An experimental study in primates. Arch. Ophthalmol. 98:1823, 1980.

122. Horwitz, J. A., Dawson, W. W., and Rubin, M. L.: Transscleral stimulator for the visual-evoked response. Am. J. Ophthalmol. 76:395, 1973.

123. LeGrand, Y.: *Light, Colour and Vision*. London, Chapman & Hall, 1957.

124. Tolentino, F. I., Freeman, H. M., Schepens, C. L., and Hirose, T.: Preoperative evaluation. Trans. Am. Acad. Ophthalmol. Otolaryngol. 81: OP 358, 1976.

125. Strong, P.: *Biophysical Measurements*. Beavertown, Ore., Tektronix Inc., 1973.

126. Gouras, P.: Primate retina: Duplex function of dark adapted ganglion cells. Science 147:1593, 1965.

Index